Partnering with Patients
to Reduce Medical Errors

Partnering with Patients to Reduce Medical Errors

Patrice L. Spath

Editor

Foreword by David B. Nash, M.D., M.B.A.

Health Forum, Inc.
An American Hospital Association Company
CHICAGO

press

Printed in the United States of America—02/04

Cover design by Tim Kaage

ISBN: 1-55648-314-7

Item Number: 181202

Library of Congress Cataloging-in-Publication Data

Partnering with patients to reduce medical errors / Patrice L. Spath, editor ; foreword by David B. Nash.
  p. cm.
  Includes index.
  ISBN 1-55648-314-7
  1. Medical errors—Prevention. 2. Patient participation. 3. Hospital care—Quality control. 4. Medical personnel and patient. I. Spath, Patrice.

R729.8.P37 2004
610–dc22   2003056996

This book is lovingly dedicated to my son,
Gordon Spath, a creative young man
with limitless intellectual and artistic potential.

Contents

List of Figures

About the Editor

Patrice L. Spath, B.A., RHIT, is a health information management professional with broad experience in health care quality and resource management. During the past 20 years, she has presented more than 300 educational programs on quality improvement, case management, clinical paths, outcomes management, and patient safety improvement topics. She has also authored numerous books and journal articles on these subjects.

Ms. Spath has extensive knowledge of patient safety improvement techniques. She has authored and edited several books on this topic, including *Error Reduction in Health Care: A Systems Approach to Improving Patient Safety* (Jossey-Bass/AHA Press, 2000) and the *Patient Safety Improvement Guidebook* (Brown-Spath & Associates, 2002). She can be reached at www.brownspath.com.

Ms. Spath serves on the advisory board for WebM&M, an online case-based journal and forum on patient safety and health care quality sponsored by the Agency for Healthcare Research and Quality (http://webmm.ahrq.gov).

About the Contributors

Kay Beauregard, R.N., M.S.A., is administrative director of Royal Oak Beaumont Hospital, Royal Oak, Michigan. The Beaumont Hospitals in Royal Oak and Troy were finalists for the 2003 American Hospital Quest for Quality Prize.

Maggie M. Finkelstein, Esquire, is an attorney in private practice affiliated with the law practice of Stevens & Lee, Lancaster, Pennsylvania. She specializes in health law and litigation.

Joel Mattison, M.D., FACS, a board-certified plastic and reconstructive surgeon, is medical director of clinical resource management at St. Joseph's Hospital in Tampa, Florida. Dr. Mattison established and edits *Off the Record,* a monthly newsletter intended to improve communication among physicians at the hospital.

David B. Nash, M.D., M.B.A., FACP, is The Dr. Raymond C. and Doris N. Grandon Professor of Health Policy and Medicine at Jefferson Medical College of Thomas Jefferson University in Philadelphia. He is also associate dean and director of the Office of Health Policy and Clinical Outcomes at Thomas Jefferson University.

Michelle H. Pelling, M.B.A., R.N., is a health care management consultant and president of The ProPell Group, Newberg, Oregon (www.propellgroup.com). She is the author of *Hospital Manager's Guide to Joint Commission Standards* and coauthor of *Outcomes Management: Using Data to Improve Decision Making.*

Thomas C. Royer, M.D., is president and chief executive officer of CHRISTUS Health, a Catholic health care system consisting of 40 hospitals and long-term care facilities in Texas, Arkansas, Louisiana, Oklahoma, Utah, and Mexico. The system is headquartered in Irving, Texas.

James W. Saxton, Esquire, is an attorney in private practice affiliated with the law practice of Stevens & Lee, Lancaster, Pennsylvania, where he is cochair of the firm's Health Law Group and chair of the Health Care Litigation Group. Mr. Saxton is also chair of the American Health Lawyers Association's Liability Practice Group.

Paula S. Swain, R.N., M.S.N., CPHQ, FNAHQ, is director of clinical and regulatory review at Presbyterian Hospital in Charlotte, North Carolina. She is also president of Swain and Associates, a firm specializing in health care quality improvement and compliance consulting and training (www.snaconsulting.com).

Steven Winokur, M.D., is medical director, quality improvement, and chief patient safety officer at Royal Oak Beaumont Hospital, Royal Oak, Michigan. The Beaumont Hospitals in Royal Oak and Troy were finalists for the 2003 American Hospital Quest for Quality Prize.

Foreword

David B. Nash, M.D., M.B.A.

Since the publication of the landmark Institute of Medicine (IOM) report *To Err Is Human: Building a Safer Health System* in 1999, it has become socially acceptable to discuss many aspects of patient safety in public. Yet, paradoxically, the principal party missing from the cacophony of voices about patient safety has been the patient. Essentially, consumers have not been invited to be partners in patient safety because no one has ever thought to ask.

Enter Patrice Spath, an accomplished author and editor, and her colleagues in their book *Partnering with Patients to Reduce Medical Errors*. Patrice Spath and her colleagues have asked the question and answered it with skill and grace.

Surely, many potential readers of this book have read recent headlines and can recite from memory some of the more egregious cases of system failure in hospitals around the nation: the overdose of chemotherapy at the Dana Farber in Boston, the tragic oxygen tank missile during an MRI in New York, the unfathomable blood transfusion mix-up at Duke Medical Center. Regrettably, the list goes on and on. And the lay press has finally picked up the gauntlet with regard to improving patient safety. Many of us remember the recent cover story in *Consumer Reports* titled "How Safe Is Your Hospital" or the *Reader's Digest* cover story "Avoiding Fatal Hospital Mistakes." It seems as though all of a sudden everyone is on guard for system failure and its terrible consequences.

I think everyone should approach this volume with the notion that we will all be patients sooner or later. I, for one, have been radicalized by my own work in this field and by a recent hospitalization for spinal fusion surgery. I wish I had had access to *Partnering with*

Patients before my own hospitalization. I cobbled together a check-list of my own design, making sure, for example, that visitors, whether nurses or colleagues, washed their hands and announced their intentions ahead of time. I was fortunate in that my physician wife was able to sleep on a cot next to my hospital bed as additional vigilance against medical error. I have tried hard to work with my own patients and physician trainees at all levels to instill the concepts of system failure and resulting medical error. But my home-grown checklist pales in comparison to the outstanding advice offered by Spath's colleagues throughout this book.

Naysayers will discount the work of Spath and her colleagues, wrapping themselves in the atavistic shroud of white coat profes-sionalism. These naysayers will claim, as researchers recently reported in the *New England Journal of Medicine*, that "most error is the result of a person unaccountable for his or her own actions; after all, we still put erasers on pencils, and errors are bound to occur no matter what systems we put in place to prevent them."

Those who are fortunate enough to read this book will gain a deeper and richer understanding of the etiology of medical error and a blueprint to participate in error prevention and reduction. I am reminded of the popular bumper sticker from the height of the Vietnam war that said, "If you are not a part of the solution, you're automatically a part of the problem."

Patrice Spath and her colleagues beg an important question: Is every patient ready, willing, and able to play a role in the drama involved in reducing medical error and improving patient safety? I would heartily answer in the affirmative, and this book will give even the faint at heart the necessary skill set to be an active and effective participant. I am confident, based on my own work and personal experience, that this challenge can be effectively met.

My own son related a story to me concerning the patient's role in patient safety at an overnight camp. Picture breakfast in a large, open, rustic cafeteria early in the morning on the banks of the Chesapeake Bay in rural Maryland. The camp "nurse" is dispensing the various medications in small Dixie cups for the scores of campers with asthma, seasonal allergies, diabetes, attention deficit disorder, and dozens of other chronic conditions endemic in our pediatric population. My 11-year-old dutifully takes his Dixie cup one morning but recognizes that his daily allergy pill somehow looks different today. He politely points this out to the dispenser, who admonishes him to take his medication and not slow up the process. Undaunted and, I hope, with my voice ringing softly in his ears, he appropriately tells the nurse, "I'm not going to take this pill because it does not look like my allergy medication." Sure enough, it was another camper's Ritalin!

Spath and her colleagues outline clever tools that we should teach to every medical, nursing, and pharmacy student in all of our schools of professional education across the nation. Imagine what it would be like for patients to be guided through a patient-centered preoperative checklist as part of the current informed consent procedure. Maybe one day, as a result of the work of Spath and others, we won't even need a book like this because socially acceptable behavior will dictate direct involvement in one's medical care at all levels, from the outpatient office to the operative suite and beyond.

Until that day arrives, what will it really take to put the patient in patient safety? Regrettably, I am not sanguine that our current efforts will provide the road map that we crave. Another national prize in patient safety or another award for hospital quality will not move the culture of blame quickly enough. I do not think that a dedicated specialist in reducing medical error or even thousands of chief quality officers or chief safety officers are enough troops on the ground to capture the hearts and minds of those on the front lines of reducing medical error.

What we really need, in my view, is to change the very fabric of medical education itself at all levels across the training continuum. We ought to be asking medical students, nurses, pharmacists, and others to ask patients what is important to them and probe their fears, concerns, and questions about their care. We should promote, as Spath and her colleagues do, the notion of "nothing about me, without me" from the patient's perspective. Perhaps, if we made *Partnering with Patients to Reduce Medical Errors* required reading for everyone in our vast and complex industry, we would begin to reach that social tipping point where every patient is concerned about his or her own safety and is willing to ask the difficult questions outlined so effectively in this book. My hat is off to Spath and her colleagues. I sincerely hope that our own professional colleagues are ready to enter into a dialogue as equals with our patients.

Preface

The need to avoid errors in the provision of health services is a major concern across all sites of health care delivery. Reports from the Institute of Medicine (IOM) in 1999 and 2001 emphasized the extent of harm that results from mistakes and the gap that still exists in the quality of care that people receive compared with the quality of care the system is capable of providing. The 1999 IOM report, *To Err Is Human: Building a Safer Health System,* put patient safety squarely in the forefront of the nation's health care agenda. The second IOM report, *Crossing the Quality Chasm: A New Health System for the 21st Century,* called for a transformation of the health care system to one that is patient-centered, safe, effective, and equitable. Patient-centeredness has been described in a variety of ways. Essential to each definition is the realization that practitioners and organizations must respond to patient-identified needs and concerns and create higher levels of patient satisfaction with the care experience. The health care industry is only just starting to embrace the patient as a partner in the safety movement.

In 1998 when I began to identify contributors for the book *Error Reduction in Health Care* (Jossey-Bass/AHA Press, 2000), I had hoped to find some practitioners or organizations that were actively involving patients in safety improvement efforts. What I discovered was that patient safety efforts at that time were largely reactive—focused primarily on finding and correcting the causes of significant adverse events. The concept of proactively building safety into health service activities was beginning to take hold in some institutions; however, improvement efforts were focused on clinical process changes, not patient involvement. Even those organizations reportedly practicing patient- or family-centered care were not explicitly asking patients (or their family members) to be involved in medical error prevention. There had been no definitive research studies of the value of consumer involvement in patient safety, which may explain why those considered to be at the cutting edge of safety improvement had not yet invited patients to participate. Consequently, *Error Reduction in Health Care* contained only a few passing references to what consumers might do to reduce medical errors.

When health care professionals began to scrutinize the causes of adverse events and near misses, it became apparent that a team effort was needed to prevent safety problems. The health care team can only be as strong as its weakest link, and, unfortunately, the weakest link is often the recipient of care—the patient. Leaders in health care quality efforts started speaking out about the importance of including patients in the safety movement. Regulatory agencies and accreditation bodies collaborated on initiatives designed to create opportunities for consumer involvement in patient safety. The National Patient Safety Foundation established a Patient and Family Advisory Council to recommend strategies for developing a patient-centered culture of patient safety in health care. The Agency for Healthcare Research and Quality funded several research projects to assess the safety benefit of patient-involvement strategies. Health care professionals began to view patients as partners, and patients began to assert themselves more in health care decision making. Four years after publication of *Error Reduction in Health Care,* the environment is now ready for a book describing how to engage patients in health care safety.

Although consumers may not appreciate the technical aspects of health care, the public does have strong opinions about what constitutes a safe health care experience. The consumer's view of health services safety is covered in chapter 1. Comments obtained through interviews with patients, family members, and health care professionals illustrate the value of involving consumers in the patient safety movement. The greatest challenge may be achieving a culture of safety that welcomes patient involvement. Many health care professionals subscribe to a "culture of individual accountability" that can inhibit collaboration with patients and their family members. If active consumer involvement is one key to improving safety, practitioners must change their beliefs about accountability. Health care is so complex that every member of the health care team, including the patient, must be actively involved in preventing mistakes.

Physicians who believe that safety depends primarily on the actions of health care practitioners may not readily perceive opportunities for patients to improve health care services. Physicians' beliefs about individual accountability are shaped during education and training and reinforced by the fault-based medical liability system. In chapter 2, Dr. Joel Mattison, a plastic and reconstructive surgeon, describes how the classic medical model has suppressed the voice of health care consumers and why changes in the traditional patient-physician relationship are needed to improve patient safety. Dr. Mattison contends that patients can be involved in the safety movement if they are just given the correct information and the right tools for the job. Practitioners and organizations committed to patient-centered care have for years sought to empower patients and family members to speak up and work collaboratively with the health care team. Only recently have these efforts incorporated safety improvement strategies. Swain and Spath, authors of chapter 3, assert that engaging consumers in health care safety requires health care professionals to first understand how things look from the patient's perspective. A real-life case study illustrates why patients want to be treated like responsible adults capable of assimilating information, asking informed questions, and having reasonable expectations. Chapter 3 contains numerous strategies and techniques that can be used to teach patients how to stay safe as they navigate the confusing, and sometimes treacherous, health care system.

Involving consumers in health care safety improvement is the right thing to do; however, practitioners may find it challenging to engage patients and family members in error prevention activities. Some patients may legitimately choose not to be involved. Often, practitioners may need to overcome communication or cultural barriers. Impediments to effective patient-practitioner collaboration can also originate from the attitudes and actions of health care professionals themselves. In chapter 4 the common collaboration obstacles on both sides of the patient-practitioner partnership are described by Pelling, along with strategies for surmounting these hurdles. One of the most significant obstacles to an effective patient partnership is the health care professional's perceived threat of legal actions. Physicians, nurses, and other caregivers may be reluctant to engage patients as partners in preventing errors if such interactions will increase the risk of liability lawsuits. In chapter 5 two health law specialists, Saxton and Finkelstein, suggest that many of the liability fears associated with open and honest practitioner-patient dialogue are overstated. These attorneys describe the legal, cultural, and regulatory issues affecting information sharing and disclosure and offer suggestions for overcoming many of the perceived legal barriers.

Involving patients in the safety movement will require a concerted effort on the part of health leaders to create an environment that embraces patients as partners in service delivery. In chapter 6, Thomas Royer details his involvement in the organizationwide patient safety efforts at the more than 30 hospitals, long-term care centers, physician offices, and outpatient clinics comprising CHRISTUS Health. As president and CEO of CHRISTUS Health, Dr. Royer is committed to gaining the trust and confidence of customers through reduction of errors, as well as through patient-centered care strategies.

Royal Oak Beaumont Hospital in Royal Oak, Michigan, is one of many health care organizations committed to involving consumers in medical error prevention. In chapter 7, Beauregard and Winokur describe how the organization is putting the patient into patient safety by creating a supportive culture and providing opportunities for education and partnership. The team at the hospital has created a firm foundation of patient safety that allows for increased involvement of patients and their families. In this chapter, readers learn more about the initiatives under way to strengthen and expand this involvement.

Most Americans are getting great health care. We've got the skilled people, the technology, and the facilities to provide health care that is second to none. And yet good isn't good enough. The health care industry must learn how to engage care recipients in error prevention activities. The environment is finally right for moving this agenda forward. Of course, this is not going to be easy—if it were, it would have been done a long time ago. The challenges facing health care in solving the safety problems are complicated and the solutions sometimes controversial. The end result can be a safe and efficient health care system in which all members of the health care team, including patients, communicate effectively with each other and share responsibility for positive outcomes. What better legacy to leave our children and grandchildren?

Patrice L. Spath
Forest Grove, Oregon
August 2003

Acknowledgments

Heartfelt gratitude goes out to all the people who candidly shared their personal perspectives about patient safety and health care encounters. These varied experiences provide a new and valuable understanding of the patient's view of health service safety. Thanks for helping health care professionals gain insights that no one of us could ever fully appreciate by ourselves.

Most of all, I would like to acknowledge the helpful input, honest feedback, and never-ending encouragement of my husband, Robert Brown. Robert, I could not have done this book without your friendship and your patience.

Partnering with Patients
to Reduce Medical Errors

1

Safety from the Patient's Point of View

Patrice L. Spath, B.S., RHIT

Consumer safety is big business in America. Numerous national and state regulatory agencies and independent oversight bodies watch over the quality of products and services in an effort to ensure that consumers are protected from economic and/or physical harm. Consumer advocacy groups alert government regulators to new safety problems or dangerous products that have evaded the current systems of inspection or sanction. Consumer associations and lawyers (joined by an alliance of lawyers and politicians) often help to bring about new consumer protection laws. Professional organizations offer another layer of safety protection for consumers through the development of licensure or certification requirements, professional standards, and self-governance. All of these groups carry out the more general role of information sharing and consumer education.

Consumer materials generally fall into one of three broad categories: education, information, or promotion. Education materials are designed to help consumers understand key safety issues about a product or service. Information materials generally focus on providing safety tips, checklists, and other aids to help individuals stay safe when using a particular product or service. Promotion materials are designed primarily to sell a product, service, or image, although they may also have an educational or informational aspect. Growth of the consumer movement in the 1960s and 1970s led to the introduction of hazard warnings on consumer products ranging from household chemical cleaners to food products to major appliances. Similar cautionary warnings about consumer services soon

1

became commonplace. Consumers were taught how to make safe choices when selecting home improvement contractors, financial investment counselors, and other services.

Health Care Consumer Protection

With the establishment of a competitive health care market in 1994 and the subsequent spread of managed care, consumers began to express concerns about the quality and safety of health care services. Groups such as the Consumer Coalition for Quality Health Care were formed for the purpose of ensuring that consumers had access to a health care system that provided meaningful consumer information and choice, consumer participation, and grievance and appeals rights for individuals denied coverage or services. Horror stories about so-called "drive-thru" baby deliveries and other seemingly inappropriate cost-cutting measures led to an increasing public outcry about declining health care quality and safety. It was also during this time that consumers began to assume more personal ownership for health care quality.

The need for individual involvement in health care quality was reinforced by the "Consumer Bill of Rights and Responsibilities" issued in November 1997 by the President's Advisory Commission on Consumer Protection and Quality in the Health Care Industry.[1] In providing consumers with a set of rights and protections, the commission acknowledged that individual consumers must assume certain responsibilities. These responsibilities include playing an active role in the treatment and management of their health and asking questions of their health care providers. The commission also encouraged health care providers to communicate more clearly with patients and their families about diagnoses, treatment options, and treatment protocols.

Patient participation began with encouraging individuals to become involved in making decisions about their personal health care. It is now expanding to embrace patient and family involvement in error prevention. As this latter agenda is advanced throughout the health care industry, it is likely that some will question whether patients are capable of understanding and promoting safety and preventing errors. In other words, does the individual patient have a purposeful role in patient safety, or is the theory merely patient-centered rhetoric that will ultimately have little influence on health care safety? Health care is often technical and requires a background knowledge of medicine to understand it. Consumers may misunderstand some health care processes or take information out of context. Patients can speak from their own experiences with health services, and this expertise can be valuable from the perspective of customer satisfaction. However, will embracing the patient as an active member of the health care team yield benefits in terms of patient safety?

To address this question, let's consider another situation in which consumers have limited ability to safeguard their personal safety. An analogy to the consumer's health care experience is airline travel. Passengers on an airplane have little control over the safety of the travel event. The average airline traveler does not have a background knowledge of aeronautics nor does the traveler understand the mechanical workings of an airplane. It is unlikely the typical airplane passenger would be able to recognize or prevent the usual causes of airline accidents.[2] Yet the airline industry has acknowledged that safe air travel is a shared responsibility. Government regulators, manufacturers, members of the airline industry, and passengers are all viewed as playing a role in air safety. The following are some strategies, suggested by Boeing, that airline travelers can use to protect themselves from being injured by the effects of turbulence:

- Always wear your seat belt when seated.
- Hold on to the seat backs or overhead bins when walking in the cabin.
- Listen to all safety announcements and follow flight crew instructions.
- Be careful when opening overhead bins following turbulence.[3]

An airplane passenger doesn't have to know how to construct an airplane or use navigational equipment to be an active participant in preventing injuries during severe turbulence. If explained in lay-person terms, travelers can even figure out some of the "unknowns" of airline travel, such as what all the noises represent and what actions the pilots are accomplishing during the flight. Passengers are considered partners in air safety, and for this reason preflight and in-flight announcements to engage passengers in this role of partner are mandatory.

Slow Embrace of Consumer Involvement

Why haven't health care consumers been embraced as partners in safety as they have in other industries? Some speculate it is because health professionals have been reluctant to admit that mistakes happen; yet it is doubtful that members of other industries are any more willing to own up to errors. It is more likely that consumers have not been invited to be partners in health care safety because no one ever thought to ask. The public has customarily relied on govern-ment regulators and members of the health care industry to protect the quality and safety of health care services. The classic advice to medical professionals, *Primum non nocere* (First, do no harm), implies that the action and decision making rests in the hands of the physician, with no role for the patient.[4] Why would consumers feel the need to be involved in medical error prevention when practi-tioners promise not to knowingly harm patients and government regulators (and attorneys) punish the people or organizations that fail to live up to this promise?

What's been missing in health care are routine "preflight" and "in-flight" safety announcements—consumers have thus not felt the need or desire to be actively engaged in the safety movement. Patients are just beginning to understand they play a role in keeping themselves safe during the health care experience. A patient focus has always underpinned medical professional rhetoric but has had surprisingly little influence on the development of true patient-practitioner partnerships. Now, with the quality and safety of health care perceived to be inadequate on many counts, the traditionally passive role of the consumer is being scrutinized and questioned.

As in the airline industry, quality and safety in health care should be a shared responsibility with the consumer. Health care consumers are similar to airline passengers in that they have a limited technical understanding of the health care experience. But health care consumers, like airline passengers, can become knowledgeable safety partners. Patients and their families will choose to be involved in different ways and at different degrees of intensity. Just as some airline passengers don't perform their safety duties, some patients will remain passive and expect health care professionals to assume all accident prevention responsibilities. Patients with chronic illnesses (like frequent air travelers) may wish to become exceptionally skilled at controlling the health care experience in an effort to reduce the risk of personal harm. All health care professionals should be striving toward developing a variety of interventions and methods that allow every consumer an opportunity to participate in the patient safety movement in a way that suits her or his needs and level of commitment.

Changing the Patient-Practitioner Relationship

Many patients are keen to take some responsibility for optimizing the outcomes of the health care experience.[5] Allowing patients to fulfill this role to their satisfaction, however, will require a change in the social relationship between health care professionals and patients. Figure 1-1 illustrates the characteristics of the traditional paternalistic health care professional and the traits that must be adopted if patient-practitioner collaboration is to be fully realized.

Figure 1-1.   Old and New Concepts of the Professional Role

The Paternalistic Professional	The Collaborative Professional
• Master of knowledge and skills	• Shared learning
• Unilateral ownership of quality and safety (patient is dependent)	• Interdependent relationship (patient is empowered)
• Individual accountability	• Collective responsibility
• Detached	• Engaged

The medical profession is already beginning to redefine the relationship between physicians and patients. Members of the Medical Professionalism Project of the American Board of Internal Medicine Foundation recently published "Medical Professionalism in the New Millennium: A Physician Charter," which encompasses a set of principles to which all medical professionals can and should aspire.[6] One of the principles, patient autonomy, addresses the need for physicians to be honest with patients and empower them to make informed decisions about their treatment. The charter supports a commitment to improving quality of care and encourages physicians to work collaboratively with other professionals to reduce medical error and increase patient safety. Unfortunately, at the present time, no mention is made of partnering with patients or consumers in this effort.

Hospital organizations that are forming safety partnerships with patients and their families readily acknowledge the need for a profound cultural shift. In the words of Judith Napier, M.S.N., cochair of the Patient Safety Committee at Children's Hospitals and Clinics, Minneapolis-St. Paul, "Optimizing patient care requires creating an institutional expectation, a shared belief, that patient safety is everyone's responsibility."[7] The need for a culture change in health care is reinforced in the report *Collaborative Education to Ensure Patient Safety*, jointly published by the Council on Graduate Medical Education (COGME) and the National Advisory Council on Nurse Education and Practice (NACNEP). One of the major recommendations in the COGME-NACNEP report is that patient safety will require a significant change in the cultures that guide current medicine and nursing practices. The councils recognize that physicians and nurses will have to adjust their own practice approaches to encourage patients to become educated and to participate in their own health care.[8]

The education of health care professionals, regulation and other forms of accountability, decision making, reward systems, performance measurement, and even the very nature of patient autonomy and involvement must be rethought. Useful as it might be, inviting patients to be partners in the safety movement will amount to little more than tinkering with the old model of health care unless there are reforms in education, regulation, professionalism, and the other health care subsystems that influence quality.

What Consumers Have to Offer

The limited availability of physicians in the first third of the 19th century prompted many Americans to depend on self-care to treat recurrent illnesses. There was also a far-reaching distrust of physicians, whose painful treatments included bloodletting and violent purgatives.[9] Eventually, medical practices changed and physicians and other health professionals became more available. Somewhere in this evolution, the patient's self-responsibility for health services, as well as the voice of the health care customer, got lost. Health care became something that was done to—not with—patients.

In the early 1990s the public's trust in the health care industry began to erode again. Several factors contributed to this mistrust, including the public perception that the industry failed in self-regulation and that health care organizations were putting their own interests above those of patients and the public.[10] The well-publicized reports of unpleasant outcomes resulting from medical errors caused even further mistrust. This general mistrust persists in spite of more rigorous regulatory oversight and nationwide patient safety improvement initiatives.

With lessening confidence in the quality and safety of health services, consumers are becoming self-advocates. The regular exercise of self-advocacy has led to more discerning health care consumers, many of whom are alert to quality problems and eager to contribute to the patient safety movement.

Can Consumers Distinguish Safe Care?

The consumer's perception of health service safety is based on input from a variety of sources: personal experiences, others' personal experiences (including general beliefs handed down through generations), and the media (books, movies, documentaries, advertisements and news, either factual or fictitious, positive and negative).

Of course, the perceptions of patients or their caregivers may be inaccurate, but perception is patients' reality and will definitely influence beliefs.

The consumer's judgment about the safety of a particular health care experience is also influenced by factors more subtle than perceptions, such as neatness of the surroundings, the practitioner's demeanor, or whether caregivers appear confident. Again, the patient or caregiver may be right or totally misinformed, but when health services are needed and a decision must be made, people will use whatever information they have available. Because the consumer's assessment of patient safety is based on several factors, the same health care experience may be considered unsafe by one person and safe by another.

If consumers are to be embraced as active partners in the patient safety movement, health care professionals cannot hold to the premise that the public is not in a position to understand or judge the safety of health services. Active participation implies the sharing of information and opinions, joint problem solving, and joint responsibility. A third factor influencing consumers' opinions about the safety of health services is their understanding or belief that the health care organization is committed to providing safe health services. Unless they have some reason to believe this commitment exists, they may suspect otherwise. Listening to *and* acting on the safety concerns of consumers can go a long way toward demonstrating a provider's dedication to patient safety.

In preparing for this chapter, a number of health care consumers (patients and caregivers) were interviewed to determine their understanding of safe health care practices and what makes them feel unsafe. Some of the people surveyed have little or no medical expertise, whereas others currently work (or have worked) in the health care industry. The comments of these consumers are found in the next sections, together with some background information about the person offering the comments. The responses are not intended to represent a valid research study nor are they an adequate sampling of all health care consumers. Respondents were self-selected from the larger group of people who were invited to participate. As such, these consumers may have stronger opinions or more to say about health care safety than the average person. Even with these shortcomings, health care professionals are encouraged to take the comments to heart. All respondents have expertise based on their lived experience of illness and health services. The value of listening and acting on the comments of these consumers is best summed up in the words of Norman McLean in his book *A River Runs Through It* (University of Chicago Press, 1989): "All there is to thinking is seeing something noticeable which makes you see something you weren't noticing which makes you see something that isn't even visible."

Views on Safety from Patients

People who have been recipients of health services were asked to respond to the following question: *What would a safe health experience look and feel like to you?* The responses were influenced by several factors, including the person's age, health status, personal experiences, and convictions. To aid in interpreting the respondents' comments, some background information is provided.

Male, 49 years old, Alabama. Background: Educator in allied health professional degree program (nonclinical). Regular user of health care services as the result of a variety of chronic conditions.

Overall, a safe health experience would be one that has no negative outcomes—no mishaps, no adverse reactions to treatment or medication, no unintended harm to the patient. I would feel safe if all information regarding my previous care was always available in my chart along with my allergies, and so on. The treating physicians and nurses should understand the medications that I am on and the potential for any adverse reactions with any additionally prescribed medications. Feeling safe also means to me that I am receiving the appropriate treatment for my condition and that I am able to freely discuss the treatment being given.

Female, 47 years old, Colorado. Background: Patient advocate specializing in support services for those injured by medical errors. She describes herself as "basically a healthy person with only periodic visits to the doctor."

In order to make health care experiences safer for all concerned, there has to be communication between the doctor, the staff, and the patient. When my husband was in the hospital, his primary care physician did not see him once. It took at least three calls for the doctor to even call me back, and the urologist who did the original biopsy did not call back even after repeated calls. Let's just say this did not inspire confidence in the doctors.

Patients must be ready and willing to assume some responsibility for their medical care. They must come into the office with a list of medications they are taking and ask questions about interactions. Maybe they need to ask these questions of their druggist or contact the manufacturer of the medication.

Male, 42 years old, Pennsylvania. Background: Editor for a health care magazine. No medical expertise or health care experience. He is in good health with only sporadic physician visits.

A safe health care experience to me would be one in which the staff asked me a lot of questions and reassured me that no matter how many questions I asked, I was not bothering them. I want to know that I can ask any question I may have. Also, the staff would explain everything they were doing. For example, if they started examining my stomach, they would say, "I'm checking here because. . . ."

The safe health care experience would start at the point of making the appointment with a competent, professional scheduler who could at least understand my problem and treat it with the urgency required of the situation. If I stated that I was concerned about whatever condition I was calling about, and an appointment wasn't available for several weeks, I would expect the scheduler to tell me what options I had for being seen earlier, either by seeing another practitioner or being placed on a cancellation list.

Female, 41 years old, Georgia. Background: Product marketing manager for publishing firm. No medical expertise or health care experience. She is an average user of health care services with no chronic conditions.

My idea of a safe health care experience: Someone would call me a couple of days prior to my health service appointment to pre-register me or I would be given a phone number or Web site where I can preregister. When presenting for the appointment, I would give my name and the provider would already have all of the information necessary to care for me. The nurse would have preread my chart and know why I was there and would ask questions for clarification. If it were necessary for the practitioner to touch me, he or she would wash up in front of me so that I knew it was sanitary. The physician would spend a few minutes reading the nurses' notes and would be aware of my presenting problem before entering my room and would wash up in front of me before touching me. He would ask for clarification, examine me thoroughly, and allow time for me to ask questions and ask about treatment options. He would make a recommendation of what treatment plan he felt best but would include me in the decision-making process. If lab work or diagnostic tests were called for, the physician would make sure that I understood exactly what was going to be done and where and all of the potential side effects. The doctor would let me know if any follow-up is necessary and be specific about when I should make another appointment if one is needed.

For lab work or tests, the technicians would give a brief description of their understanding of the presenting problem and what diagnostic tests were to be performed. This would give me the opportunity to make sure that the tests being performed were the same as those the physician had told me about. The technicians would let me know how my tests and lab work were going to be processed so there was no chance that they would be misplaced or mislabeled as someone else's results. If possible, I would see my name and account number on the film, or tube, or whatever. At the conclusion of the test, I would be told when the results would be back and how to obtain them. If I were told that the doctor would contact me, then the doctor's office would call.

Anytime anyone was going to administer medication to me, he or she would state what the medication was, what it was for, and confirm that I was the person who was to receive the medication. If the person administering the medication had to touch me, he or she would wash his or her hands in front of me prior to doing so.

Female, 59 years old, New York. Background: Antique dealer and amateur artist. No medical expertise or any other health care background. She only occasionally sees a physician; however, a few years ago she cared for an elderly relative who had several chronic conditions and multiple hospital admissions.

Society has unrealistically high health care expectations. Medical accidents will happen because of human error. Not every injured, sick, or dying person will be healed, and medical accidents will happen because of human error. There must be an extensive campaign to modify the public's unrealistic expectations. If my expectations are more in line with reality, then it will be easier for me to have the perception of a safe health care experience.

In a safe health care experience, a team of health care professionals is responsible for my care. They understand that I am also a member of the team. Members of the team are accessible to me. Information is shared with me. I have input with regard to their plans for my care. Because we communicate and I am part of the process, I am not a helpless victim. I would also feel safer if I had a patient advocate to watch over my care when I'm not able to personally keep track of what's happening. Every patient needs an advocate.

Ideally, my medical history and medications are part of a centralized database of patient information that is easily accessible to my team. The team responsible for my care is not sleep deprived. If they work long hours without sufficient rest, their decision-making abilities could be impaired and my safety will be jeopardized.

Male, 59 years old, South Carolina. Background: Higher education professor and education design specialist. He is a member of a hospital governing board.

I would feel safe if I received a quality diagnosis that was offered by a reputable professional and concurred with by at least two or three other professional opinions. My health care providers would need to be fully certified or accredited and technically proficient. Staff caring for me should take the time to explain and respond to my concerns and be spiritually enlightened. My surroundings should be aesthetically pleasing, and my family members and other significant individuals (clergy, attorney) should have appropriate access to me.

The last consideration in my safety would be adequate follow-up procedures. This would include timely and routine checks on my progress. Also, I should be provided an opportunity to give feedback to my providers and be encouraged to make suggestions for improving health care services.

Male, 56 years old, Georgia. Background: Health care journalist; no clinical background. He has Type II diabetes requiring periodic outpatient visits.

Every medical experience I have is colored by the fact that I have Type II diabetes. Accordingly, the first thing that would make me feel safe with health care professionals would be the fact that they knew my history and that they were well versed in all aspects of the disease. I would expect to be asked what my latest blood sugars are, how I am feeling, and what I am doing in terms of diet and exercise. My physical examination should include tests specifically designed to assess possible complications from diabetes (retinopathy, circulation problems, etc.).

I feel safe with a health care provider when he or she seems genuinely concerned about my well-being and willing to listen to me and answer my questions. I also feel safe with an individual who seems confident, knowledgeable, and honest about the possible side effects of any drugs I may need to take or any procedure about to occur. Honesty, openness, caring, concern, and knowledge—these are what inspire my confidence and make me feel safe.

Views on Safety from Caregivers

A study funded by CareThere.com estimates that more than one-quarter (26.6 percent) of the adult population in the United States has provided care for a chronically ill, disabled, or aged family member or friend.[11] Based on current census data, that translates into more than 50 million people. Many caregivers provide full-time care for a family member or friend and deal with a wide array of medical conditions and diagnoses. The caregiver's perception of health care safety is significantly influenced by the experiences shared with his or her spouse, parent, children, sibling, or friend. People serving as caregivers offer a perspective on safety that is different from that of the patient's. To gain the caregiver's point of view for this chapter, members of the National Family Caregivers Association were invited to respond to the question: *What would a safe health experience for your loved one look and feel like to you?*

Female, 45 years old, Texas. Background: Caregiver for her husband, who suffered a stroke and kidney failure about 10 years ago. She has a degree in chemistry and biology but has not worked in the health care industry.

Here are my suggestions for making the health care experience safer for patients:

1. Chairs (dialysis chairs, wheelchairs, and so on) and stretchers used for patients who may be physically incapacitated should *always* have locks on the wheels and should always be locked for patient transfer.
2. Staff should always communicate with patients and/or their family members as to the patient's abilities, discomforts, aches, and disabilities *before* moving them. They should continue to check on the patient's level of comfort as they proceed.
3. Contact information should be posted prominently so that patients, family members, and even employees can easily inform the appropriate building personnel of safety concerns.
4. Listen to the concerns of patients and their family members. Physicians and other staff should appreciate that when patients or family members bring up safety concerns, they view the

issues as real problems and are only trying to help the professionals do their job better and keep themselves or their loved ones safe.

5. Physicians and other staff should understand that when patients or family members request certain medications, tests, or other treatments, they often know what they are talking about. A physician or nurse who may have only just met the patient can't know as much as the patient who has the chronic condition or a family member who has been caring for that person.

6. Most of all, health care professionals should remember that they are human and will make mistakes. There is no harm in checking with the patient or family members for a second opinion. And there is no excuse for ignoring or trivializing patient input. Emotional security is just as important to the patient as physical safety. Last, staff members should also keep in mind that patients are human. They are not machines or slabs of meat to throw on a table to poke and prod. Patients are not insignificant; they are human beings who need your help.

Female, 41 years old, New Jersey. Background: Caregiver for her 11-year-old daughter who has multiple chronic conditions, including kidney disease (renal agenesis, renal dysplasia, Grade IV bilateral vesicoureteral reflux), and autism (Asperger syndrome).

A "safe experience" would be one in which I know a procedure is being done properly with no hesitation on the part of the professional and minimal discomfort for my child. That said, I think that family caregivers need to be present at all times, educated about medical procedures, and be vigilant observers. I've had a few instances where errors occurred even in my presence:

- A pediatric nurse tried to use an adult-size catheter on my infant daughter. I stopped her. I happened to know it was the adult size because I had been hospitalized during my pregnancy and was catheterized several times. I called a doctor in to perform the procedure.
- The laboratory did not check my daughter's immunization records and gave her an extra hepatitis B shot. The error wasn't

noticed until I pointed out on the chart that she had already received three shots. If they'd had me sign a consent form (as was usual), the mistake might have been noticed before the injection was given. My daughter is a medically fragile child who previously went into shock after a DPT immunization.

- During an MRI, the portion of my daughter's spine being checked for tethered cord due to spina bifida occulta was not well supported as she was coming out of anesthesia.
- While my daughter was under anesthesia for the MRI, no one even thought to put a pull-up diaper on her so I had to do it. She has enuresis due to her kidney disease.

Views on Safety from Health Care Professionals

Although patient safety is a shared commitment among all health care professionals, many are not certain of how to go about effectively involving consumers in the safety movement. Practitioners' training and work experiences significantly influence their patient safety beliefs. To broaden the views of health care professionals, a physician and nurse were asked to respond to the question: *What would the health care experience be like if patients and families were actively involved in making health care safer?*

Male, pediatrician, Ohio. After retiring from an active practice, he worked as vice president for medical affairs in two hospitals and as a part-time medical director for a health plan. At the present time he consults with several health care organizations to address such issues as JCAHO and regulatory compliance, physician practice management, medical staff administration and reorganization, and physician education in medical staff functions and responsibilities.

A safe health care experience is one in which there is effective communication between patients and physicians. Unfortunately, for the most part, physician-patient contact has yet to become a true interactive exchange of information with both parties striving to reach a mutually satisfactory care goal. Physicians by training, or because of perceived time constraints, frequently present a closed attitude to patients. Sensing this, patients are often intimidated from actively participating in their care. When patients are passive participants, they don't volunteer information and refrain from asking questions. In this circumstance, neither the physician nor the patient receives the information and understanding necessary for a safe health care experience.

Physicians have to accept that patients come armed with more information from outside, albeit not necessarily always reliable, sources. Patients want to discuss that information with the physician. Physicians must take the lead in presenting an environment where the patient feels free to exchange information and cooperate with, or challenge, the diagnostic plan or the course of treatment. The physician's people skills have to be honed to match his or her technical skills.

To create a more satisfying patient-practitioner relationship, physicians must allow interchange to occur and must respect the patient's desire and right to question and challenge. It must come to be accepted that this type of relationship is not, by definition, confrontational. The increasing complexity of patient care demands this type of patient-physician interaction. When patients have a better understanding of their condition and treatment, they can become the first line of defense against misadventures and unsafe situations.

Female, registered nurse, California. She has 25 years of health care experience as a critical care nurse and a certified health care quality professional. For the past eight years she has been on the "patient side" of health care, having suffered a spinal cord injury, which resulted in quadriplegia. Two years after her injury, she was diagnosed with breast cancer. She describes herself as "an experienced inpatient," having had three hospitalizations for a total of four weeks, two months in acute rehab, and four surgical procedures.

Patients are much more likely to perceive their health care experience as safe when they are included as active participants rather than treated as helpless victims. Patients should be encouraged to participate as fully as possible in their care. From my perspective as both a nurse and a patient, the following suggestions are offered to physicians, nurses, and other health care professionals:

- Actively listen to your patients' questions, concerns, and observations. As a patient, I feel safer when I perceive staff to be listening to me.
- Encourage patients to ask questions or provide input to their care whenever you are with them for whatever reason. Patients don't feel safe if the only way they can get the caregiver's attention is by using their call light or lodging a complaint.
- Teach those patients who are coherent and interested everything that is reasonable for them to know. Teaching should be done verbally with the same instructions and information provided in writing.
- Encourage your patients to notify you or another staff member if they believe something is "not right" or "abnormal."
- Teach those patients with an expressed desire to know (just ask first) how to be observant for problems and when to call for assistance (for example, IV line or injection site concerns, what the alarms mean, what should occur when an IV bottle is empty, when to be concerned about a dressing, and so on).
- Give a medication sheet to coherent hospitalized patients and crosscheck the medications with the patients before administration (including IVs). This collaboration is also a good time to teach safe medication administration practices to patients. Provide patients with brief written descriptions of any new medications, similar to the instruction sheets that outpatient pharmacies provide to customers.
- Tell patients about the hand-washing policy. Ask them to speak up if practitioners entering the room fail to wash their hands before touching them.
- Provide mechanisms for your patients to share suggestions for improving the overall health care experience (ways to do things that are safer, smarter, quicker, less costly) and ideas for making their own care better. When patients are able to share their views, they are more likely to be satisfied, and a satisfied patient feels safer.

The caveat to these recommendations is that communication must be free flowing and two-way. Caregivers must establish relationships with their patients, even if very short term, and must be good listeners. In a safe environment, caregivers are confident, competent, communicative, and comfortable with their patients. They listen to their patients' concerns and ideas with sincere interest and then do what they say they will do to follow through. This may involve further communications with the patient, communications with other health care professionals, timely intervention, documentation, or reporting. To me, this makes for the best "feel safe" care.

Implications for Patient Safety

As the role of the health care consumer in patient safety receives increased attention, it is important to consider the opinions and preferences of patients and their families. Several primary themes can be found in the comments of those people participating in the formal interviews. Consumers want practitioners to treat patients with care, compassion, and honesty. They want practitioners to have a broader understanding of patients, one that takes into consideration the emotional, social, mental, spiritual, and physical dimensions of the person's medical condition. Patients want to be listened to and respected for their opinions. Patients, caregivers, and practitioners alike emphasized the importance of involving patients as part of the care team and teaching them what they can do to keep themselves safe. Despite the limitations of this informal survey process, the results are consistent with other studies of health care consumer preferences.[12]

Francine R. Gaillour, M.D., speculates that the trend toward active patient participation could lead to the emergence of a new medical specialty: the patient advocate.[13] According to Dr. Gaillour, the physician serving as a patient advocate would not provide any direct care; rather, he or she would play the role of translator of medical knowledge and facilitator of treatment decision making, helping the client sort through diagnosis, treatment, and care options. A patient advocate role, whether assumed by a physician, nurse, or other knowledgeable health care professional or layperson, could improve patient safety. For this reason, the National

Patient Safety Foundation (NPSF) is committed to educating people about how a patient advocate can help health care safety. The NPSF brochure, "Role of the Patient Advocate," offers tips for patients in choosing an advocate to look out for their best health care interests.[14]

Learning about Safety from Patients

Health care professionals are learning to value the expertise of patients, and many are eager to tap into a patient's experience to learn what can be done to improve the safety of health care. The National Patient Safety Agency (NPSA) in the United Kingdom is actively involving patients in several health service safety initiatives. In late 2002, the NPSA initiated a study to determine the root causes of problems surrounding the use of infusion devices to deliver fluids and drugs to patients. The NPSA researchers reviewed the global evidence on infusion device user errors, looked at best practices already taking place in the National Health Services, sought feedback from health professionals, and interviewed patients who had used a pump in the hospital for chemotherapy, pain control, or insulin control. The patient interviews elicited a great deal of information on what being on a pump feels like from the patient's viewpoint as well as many valid safety concerns. Study findings that concentrate on safety issues relevant to nurses and nursing care are presented in the appendix at the end of this chapter.[15]

Involving Patients on the Health Care Team

Safety is a system property that has yet to be achieved in health care. A safe system is one in which the entire system is designed to prevent errors and minimize the effects of ordinary human mistakes. By involving the patient as a member of the health care team, several pairs of eyes, each with a different perspective, can help make the system of care safer. Different members of the team may see red flags or opportunities at times and places that no single member of the team is in a position to see. A certain amount of good redundancy is built into the system when everyone is on the alert for mistakes. Health care processes must be made transparent so that everyone (including the patient) knows what is going on and why. Health care is so complex that no single discipline or care recipient can possibly maintain the situational awareness needed to prevent adverse events.

Nothing less than a revolution in medical culture may be needed to fully accept patients as legitimate members of the health care team. During his training, Dr. Marc Ringel sensed he was being constantly indoctrinated with two principles:

1. The doctor must know everything. It is not okay to say, "I don't know."
2. The doctor is to be in charge in every patient care situation. Everyone else, no matter what the expertise or knowledge of the patient, must defer to the physician.[16]

In medical school, soon-to-be physicians are not taught to be team players, and many other health care professionals fail to receive initial training in team collaboration skills.[17] Clearly, teaching health professions to act as a team must be accomplished or practitioners may never be able to fully embrace the patient as a valued team member. Although consumers may be positioned to bring about some improvements in the safety of health services, they cannot influence the curricula for doctors, nurses, and allied health professionals. It will be up to the academic community to adopt the 1998 recommendations of the Pew Commission, which urged education systems to ensure that graduates are successful in meeting the expectations of health care consumers.[18]

Patients don't want to believe that physicians, nurses, or other health care professionals make mistakes, especially when it is a caregiver they know and trust. Yet there is a growing public realization that mistakes happen and the patient (and family members or caregiver) can play a part in reducing the chance of a harmful accident. The role of patients in health care safety is not limited to providing practitioners with the information necessary to do their job. To achieve the full safety benefit from patient involvement, health care organizations must incorporate patient feedback into safety improvement initiatives, set up opportunities for dialogue between patients and health care professionals, and incorporate the patient perspective into initial training and continuing education programs for caregivers. At the patient-practitioner level, patients must be respected for the knowledge they have. This means listening and responding to patients' questions, handling problems so they don't recur, sharing information that empowers patients to prevent errors, and actively encouraging patients to be partners with the health care team. If you remain skeptical about patients' desire and ability to join the team, reread the comments from patients, family members, and health care professionals found earlier in this chapter.

The degree of patient participation in the treatment process depends on their physical and mental condition, willingness, knowledge, and experience. Yet patients always have some role in achieving a satisfactory outcome by committing to treatment, becoming educated enough to participate in the healing process, and being cooperative and compliant during and after care delivery. To play even a minor role in the patient safety movement, consumers must be taught how to communicate effectively with health care practitioners.

Raising the safety performance of a complex system like health care means recognizing that it is the people on the frontlines that have to make and sustain change. Safe results every time cannot be mandated by regulatory agencies or organizational leaders. Rather, the focus must be on building the capacity of each member of the health care team to identify problems and improve the system. Every member of the team, including the patient, must be empowered to speak up and work collaboratively.

References

1. Advisory Commission on Consumer Protection and Quality in the Health Care Industry. "Appendix A. Consumer Bill of Rights and Responsibilities," in *Quality First: Better Health Care for All Americans* (1998) [http://www.hcqualitycommission.gov/final/append_a.html]. Accessed July 2003.

2. Common causes of airplane accidents: (1) failure to adequately compensate for wind conditions during takeoff and climb out; (2) takeoff in wind conditions beyond the pilot's or airplane's capabilities; (3) engine failure or loss of power after takeoff; (4) failure to maintain adequate airspeed during takeoff and climb out, resulting in a departure stall; (5) attempting takeoff with too strong a tailwind component; (6) failure to compensate for high-density altitude conditions or attempting takeoff in density altitude conditions beyond the airplane's capabilities; and (7) improper configuration of the aircraft for weight and flight conditions. From J. K. Boatman, "Plan the Takeoff—And Take Off According to the Plan," *AOPA Pilot* (June 2001).

3. Boeing, "What Can Passengers Do—Enhancing Your Air Travel Safety" [http://www.boeing.com/commercial/safety/pf/pf_passenger_role.html. Accessed July 2003.

4. J. D. Shelton, "The Harm of 'First, Do No Harm,'" *Journal of the American Medical Association* 284, no. 21 (2000): 2687–88.

5. D. B. Nash and others, *Connecting with the New Healthcare Consumer: Defining Your Strategy* (New York: Aspen Publishers, 2001).

6. Medical Professionalism Project, American Board of Internal Medicine Foundation, "Medical Professionalism in the New Millennium: A Physician Charter," *Annals of Internal Medicine* 136, no. 3 (2002): 243–46.

7. L. Harteker, "Partnerships for Patient Safety: Profiles of Four Hospitals," *Advances in Family-Centered Care* (January–June 2003): 17–26.

8. National Advisory Council on Nurse Education and Practice and the Council on Graduate Medical Education, *Collaborative Education to Ensure Patient Safety,* a report to the Secretary, U.S. Department of Health and Human Services, and U.S. Congress (December 2000) [http://bhpr.hrsa.gov/nursing/nacnep/patientsafety.htm].

9. A. Wrynn, "The History of American Health, Hygiene and Fitness," SUNY Cortland [http://personal.ecu.edu/estesst/2323/readings/americanpe.html]. Accessed July 2003.

10. S. R. Cruess, S. Johnston, and R. L. Cruess, "Professionalism for Medicine: Opportunities and Obligations," *The Medical Journal of Australia* 177, no. 4 (2002): 208–11.

11. National Family Caregivers Association Random Sample Survey of 1,000 Adults, Summer 2000 [http://www.nfcacares.org/NFC2002_stats.html]. Accessed July 2003.

12. J. Murphy and others, "The Quality of Physician-Patient Relationships: Patient Experiences 1996–1999," *Journal of Family Practice* 50, no. 2 (2001): 130–36; B. E. Landon and others, "Health Plan Characteristics and Patients' Assessment of Quality," *Health Affairs*

20, no. 2 (2001): 274–84; P. Little and others, "Preferences of Patients for Patient-Centered Approach to Consultation in Primary Care: Observational Study," *British Medical Journal* 322, no. 7284 (2001): 468–72; "The Evolving Patient Physician Relationship," *Pfizer Journal* (1998) [http://www.thepfizerjournal.com/TPJ06.pdf], accessed July 2003; A. M. Stiggelbout and G. M. Keibert, "A Role for the Sick Role: Patient Preferences Regarding Information and Participation in Clinical Decision-Making," *Canadian Medical Association Journal* 157, no. 4 (1997): 383–89; C. Edwards, "A Proposal That Patients Be Considered Honorary Members of the Healthcare Team," *Journal of Clinical Nursing* 11, no. 3 (2002): 340–48; M. Attree, "Patients' and Relatives' Experiences and Perspectives of 'Good' and 'Not so Good' Quality Care," *Journal of Advanced Nursing* 33, no. 4 (2001): 456–66.

13. F. R. Gaillour, "The 'Perfect Storm' in Healthcare: Crisis or Opportunity?" *HealthLeaders News* (January 6, 2003) [http://www.health leaders.com/news/feature1.php?contentid=40951]. Accessed July 2003.

14. National Patient Safety Foundation, "Role of the Patient Advocate" (2002) [http://www.npsf.org/download/PatientAdvocate.pdf]. Accessed July 2003.

15. A. Richardson, "Infusion Pumps: The Views of Patients." Unpublished paper prepared for the National Patient Safety Agency (May 2003).

16. M. Ringel,"Mistakes in Medicine," *Nexus* (March/April 2003) [http://www.nexuspub.com/articles/2003/march2003/zen_mar_2003.htm]. Accessed July 2003.

17. Council on Social Work Education, *Myths and Opportunities: An Examination of the Impact of Discipline-Specific Accreditation on Interprofessional Education* (Alexandria, Va.: Council on Social Work Education, 1999), 3; National Advisory Council on Nurse Education and Practice and the Council on Graduate Medical Education, *Collaborative Education to Ensure Patient Safety.*

18. E. H. O'Neil and the Pew Health Professions Commission, *Recreating Health Professional Practice for a New Century,* The Fourth Report of the Pew Health Professions Commission (San Francisco: Center for the Health Professions at the University of California, December 1998).

Infusion Pumps:
The Views of Patients*

Ann Richardson

Research Methodology

This research by the National Patient Safety Agency (NPSA) was limited to patients who had used an infusion pump during a stay in a hospital within the past five years for pain or symptom control following an investigation, treatment, or surgery; chemotherapy; intravenous feeding; or insulin control because they were diabetics. All participants were recruited through organizations for people with cancer or diabetes, either via a mailing to members about the research or through local support group organizers. Some were found by word of mouth from other research participants.

A short description of the nature and purpose of the study was prepared for those to be interviewed. They were assured that the information would be treated as confidential and that their treatment would not be affected by a decision to take part. A topic guide was used, covering the experiences of patients from their initial use of an infusion pump to the point of completion. The interviews were tape-recorded and transcribed verbatim. The information collected was carefully analyzed as a whole and by type of use. A copy of the research report was subsequently sent to all people interviewed for their comments.

*Unpublished paper prepared for the National Patient Safety Agency, United Kingdom, May 2003, and reprinted here by permission of the agency. Ann Richardson is patient experience and public involvement project manager, National Patient Safety Agency, London, England.

In all, 24 interviews were carried out, 13 in person and 11 by telephone. The participants were 7 men and 17 women, ranging in age from the early 20s to late 70s. In terms of diagnosis, 16 had cancer (or, in one case, a woman whose husband had died from cancer), 7 were people with diabetes (including 1 mother of a child with diabetes), and 1 had an unclear diagnosis. Of those with cancer, most had used a pump for more than one purpose: 13 for chemotherapy, 11 for morphine or other painkiller following an operation, and 3 for other purposes, such as intravenous feeding. The numbers involved in these respective categories were not purposively sought but simply emerged from the process of recruitment.

Study Results

Understanding the Infusion Pump

Almost all participants thought that it was important to understand as much as possible about their treatment, including the infusion pump. But there was considerable variation in the extent to which they were informed. Most of those having chemotherapy said that nurses tended to provide a lot of information while setting up the pump ("That's your time with them, when you have an opportunity to talk about it all"). Although much of this discussion centered on the drugs and their side effects, those who wanted information about the pump generally felt able to ask for it, with nurses ready to answer questions. On the other hand, a few would have liked to have had information earlier, because the first day of chemotherapy was "not a good day to ingest that information."

In contrast, those who used a pump for pain relief were often given little information or given it at the wrong time. A number said they could not remember being told anything about the pump but knew they must have been given some information because they understood the mechanics of controlling the dosage via the booster button. Some explicitly remembered a discussion about this. A few said they were given no information at all and felt quite shocked to wake up and find themselves attached to a pump. It was agreed that it could be difficult to find the right time for a discussion, as patients had other worries immediately before an operation and were too drowsy afterward.

The role of the booster button in the use of morphine was an issue on which clearer information was felt by patients to be particularly important. Two participants were hesitant to use their morphine fully for fear of addiction. One woman was very worried that the supply might run out and therefore tended to underdose herself ("I was very nervous of using up my quota and then not having pain relief for a long time afterward").

Participants were asked about the extent to which they had been informed about safety issues concerning the pump, such as the alarms, batteries, or need to avoid mobile phones; virtually no one could remember having been given any such details. Some said that they had seen notices about not using mobile phones because it could affect the equipment but were not clear about the details ("We were never told *which* equipment. I thought it was for people on ventilators").

Supervision of the Pump

Most participants believed that their pump was well supervised. Nurses were said to be "quite vigilant" and responded fairly quickly when alarms went off, especially for those on chemotherapy. But some people were less content with the speed of nursing attention, particularly those using a pump for pain control, where alarms were often not attended to quickly. Some said they had little sense that anyone was watching what was happening, and some had waited a long period for help. One woman, whose morphine had run out, said she was left for several hours in pain.

Because of the apparent difficulties of getting nurses' attention, a number of patients spoke of doing as much as they could for themselves, and one tried to help others. One woman indicated that she watched the nurses carefully and learned to adjust the pump for herself. Another spoke about the importance of mutual help by patients: "It's a terrifying scenario. The hospital relies on patients taking as much interest in each other as do the staff. You just pray to God that someone would help you if you ran into difficulties."

But some people thought it was potentially dangerous for patients to get involved in technical aspects of the pump.

Practical Problems

Patients tended to have strong views about the cannula. Many commented that it was very painful to insert and that nurses often did not get it right the first time. Some nurses were much more successful than others ("There were one or two that had the knack"); it was particularly worrisome to patients when nurses got flustered or panicky in an unsuccessful attempt. Patients varied in their willingness to refuse treatment from what they believed to be the less competent staff, whereas a number wished to and some did, and at least one did not refuse because she did not want to give offense.

A few people spoke of being pleasantly surprised when a cannula was inserted easily. In one case, for instance, a nurse used a very small needle with much reduced pain, and the patient then wondered why these were not used all the time ("Had they ordered all these particular sizes, and they had to be used?"). Another patient found that one nurse used a better location for the insertion, making it not at all painful.

Many participants disliked the physical restrictions imposed by a cannula. One man described lying in bed "like a statue" at first because of fear of pulling it out. Others talked about the difficulty of performing ordinary tasks, such as getting out of bed, eating, or reading, when one needed to move the hand and arm. The pulling of the needle entailed in such activity could be the source of some anxiety ("You feel that prick and you think maybe it's gone through the wall of the vein or something").

A number of patients found the pump's movable stand to be awkward to maneuver, especially over stepped areas or through doors, and they were conscious of needing to take great care not to trip over the wires ("It's a complete art form being able to walk around with one of those—any cancer survivor's a Fred Astaire by the end of it"). Some people commented that moving around involved a lot of palaver, sometimes because an alarm would go off accidentally and sometimes because of the sheer amount of equipment involved ("Everything came with you—you went up and down these stairs looking like something from Venus"). But most participants learned to move around over time and some never found moving to be a problem.

Emotional Needs and Support

Perhaps most strikingly, a number of patients spoke about their often neglected emotional needs associated with the pump. They stressed that finding themselves in need of such treatment was itself difficult, and the pump only served to underline the seriousness of their situation: "Faced with these pumps and things, emotionally it was a big shock. . . . I could see my life changing. You never think you're going to have to be wired up to one of these machines and have drugs pumped into you."

But the pump itself gave rise to considerable anxiety, often because of misunderstandings about how it worked. For instance, a common source of worry was seeing air bubbles in the tube, as people had understood from television programs that air bubbles in their bloodstream were dangerous ("The first time I saw an air bubble, I remember being totally petrified. I thought, 'Right, that is it—you are a goner!'"). A similar concern was seeing blood backed up into the pump, which several people found disquieting.

Moreover, some people intensely disliked the sense of being attached to a piece of equipment. It gave them a feeling of being "tethered" ("It's like being a prisoner with a ball and chain around your foot. . . . I felt quite claustrophobic at times"). One woman noted that this did not matter so much when she was ill but was irritating as she became better. One man found it disconcerting that the pump faced away from him, as he felt himself connected to an "alien" thing; this fear would have been eased if he could have seen it.

Perhaps the most worrying event was hearing the alarm attached to an infusion pump, especially the first time. This was not only very annoying ("It could go wrong eight times in a night—you'd be just going back to sleep and it would bleep again; sometimes I felt like throwing the machine out of the window"), but it could also be a source of real panic among those who assumed that it indicated a crisis. Moreover, the fact that the alarms went off frequently raised a fundamental issue of patient safety, because everyone began to ignore them: "The alarm is almost more redundant than a burglar alarm in a house with the neighbors ignoring it—imagine, if there had been a *real* problem here and we were just ignoring it."

The emotional responses of a few patients, it might be added, were more positive. Two said that they came to view the pump as a "friend" because it was providing important pain relief or treatment.

Safety

This study was commissioned with an interest in patient safety, and participants recounted a number of incidents, most of which arose from human error. Two patients had their lines severely pulled on or pulled out accidentally; one line got caught in a vacuum cleaner and another was pulled out by a nurse while the pump was being rigged up ("It was extraordinarily painful; I just had surgery that morning"). One woman's Hickman line was wrongly unscrewed one night so that it fell apart onto the floor the next morning. After 15 seconds during which the patient couldn't breathe, the nurse managed to screw it back again. The same woman also suffered a nurse's trying to flush an antibiotic into the line neat rather than diluted. Fortunately, her husband noted that something seemed wrong and stopped the procedure.

One woman believed that her diabetic daughter was put at risk because of ignorance about diabetes on the part of the nursing staff. Soon after setting up an insulin pump, the nurses asked her about the appropriate rate ("One nurse seemed to think that if the blood sugar was low, you needed more insulin; she had it totally the wrong way around—and that was scary"). A possible seizure was averted only because an endocrinologist happened to be on the ward and adjusted the pump appropriately.

A few experiences arose from nurses' apparently not concentrating on the matter at hand. One patient experienced an inaccurately inserted cannula and as a result was burned by chemotherapy drugs. Another had antisickness drugs put into the cannula in the wrong direction because a nurse was chatting with someone. Another patient found that her chemotherapy was not going through because the nurse had set the pump incorrectly. Two people had regular difficulties reaching their call button; one wife noted that nurses placed it out of reach every time they made her husband's bed.

One patient was highly concerned about a general lack of cleanliness, stating that nurses didn't wash their hands between patients and that the hospital itself was very unclean. It had been stressed to her that she should be kept very clean because of her neutropenia, yet the ward was quite dirty: "They give you advice about keeping clean, keeping away from animals, and instructing you to live in sterile conditions. And you're sitting in a ward watching cockroaches going across the floor, and you pick up dirt like you wouldn't believe. All the wards are splattered with blood, and the toilets weren't clean."

None of the patients had lodged a formal complaint about safety concerns presumably because of a reluctance to be a bother or to single out one nurse among an otherwise good team. There was also a concern about the possible consequences of rocking the boat: "When you've got to be there all the time, you don't want to fall out with any nurse or put any blame on anybody. Obviously, all the nurses stick together. And you hope it won't happen again."

Other Nursing Issues

A major concern for a number of participants was an apparent lack of knowledge among nurses about infusion pumps. The patients were disconcerted by the nurses' own hesitancies: "It was two [nurses] fumbling about that didn't seem to know what they were doing; they were saying, 'Do you think this is right?' and 'I'm not sure about this'—and you're thinking 'Oh, dear.'"

The handling of morphine was also an issue. One large man who found that the normal dose of morphine had limited effect after a major operation was distressed that nurses were unable to alter his dose, and he had to wait for a doctor. Three participants felt that they had become addicted to morphine. Although none blamed this on the nursing staff, they argued that the subsequent withdrawal of morphine was not handled well ("They just took it off and took it away and that was that"). Indeed, two suffered severe withdrawal symptoms, one on a regular basis because she was in and out of the hospital frequently ("I suffered cold turkey every time I came out of hospital without really knowing why").

A number of comments were offered about the general nursing care. Some patients couldn't praise nurses highly enough ("They were very, very caring—absolutely brilliant, cheerful, and positive"). But many participants noted that the nurses were overworked and stressed. Although some patients were sympathetic to the difficulties, others felt less so, especially when the nurses themselves were moody. One man aptly summarized the general problem: "The good nurses are run off their feet, whereas the others are standing around talking."

Coming Off the Pump

Coming off the pump was generally a fairly straightforward experience. Most people said that they knew what was happening, although there was little explanation ("They just came along and disconnected it"). Several spoke of the sense of release when they came off the pump ("It's the biggest relief you can imagine—you are free again"). Two people found it annoying that the cannula was not removed until just before they left the hospital, although they could see the reason for it. Few people felt there were problems associated with the removal of the cannula, but one man said removing the associated tape was painful.

Issues for Diabetic Regular Insulin Pump Users

The participants who were regular insulin pump users raised completely different issues. For them, the principal problem was not coming to terms with new equipment but rather getting the hospital staff to allow them to use their own pump while they were in the hospital. Four patients had managed to do so and were very appreciative of this decision ("It was very much a case of 'you know what to do with your pump, so if you're happy, we won't mess about in any way, unless there is an emergency'"). In most cases, the use of the patient's own pump had been preceded by some discussion between the patient and hospital staff, sometimes with considerable resistance from some staff.

These patients were concerned, however, about the ability of hospital staff to cope with their pumps (for instance, if they were under an anesthetic) because of a lack of familiarity with the pumps. Several patients brought detailed written information together with the phone number for a diabetes support team. But they did note an eagerness to learn ("I had everybody and their granny coming to look at it. . . . I had to tell them what I was doing and why I was doing it. They were all fascinated").

On five separate occasions, one participant had been required to use hospital equipment during her operation. She ascribed this to ignorance on the part of hospital staff, but she intensely disliked having decisions made for her ("It's not even a discussion between yourself and the doctors—it's 'you do what they say' and that's it").

Conclusions and Recommendations

Probably the most common recommendation among the research participants was for better training for nurses on how to work with and around infusion pumps. It was suggested that this should apply to all nurses, even those who would not normally handle a pump, so they could know how to cope in an emergency.

Some of this training should be on technical matters. Nurses should be trained to check that pumps are functioning properly so that they are not found to be faulty at the last minute. Nurses should also ensure that patients on pumps always have access to their call button (for instance, by looping the cord over the patient's hand). One woman, who had worked in television, spoke of a rule that no one ever stepped across a camera operator's cable and suggested there should be a similar rule about not stepping over any line connecting patients to equipment. The diabetic participants on regular insulin pumps argued that nursing staff needed to gain more familiarity with these pumps, possibly through more focused discussions with users.

More attention to the emotional needs of patients was thought to be equally important. Participants indicated that nurses should understand that being on a pump is an unusual experience, and patients may require considerable reassurance. Nurses also need to understand patients' fears concerning pumps and should be trained to appreciate a patient's sense of confinement. Two people suggested that nurses should be required to experience this for a day or two ("just to see what it's like").

Many participants stressed the need for fuller information about their disease and treatment. This information should also be imparted to the main caregiver whenever possible. It should include information about the pump—why patients were having one, how it operates, how long patients would be having it, the dosage, likely problems, and the details of its use. Participants also suggested that patients be given ample warning about issues likely to worry them, such as air bubbles and the alarms. A system for collecting and disseminating ideas from patients on how to cope with a pump would be helpful.

This early research by the NPSA serves as a good indicator of the benefit of listening to patients' views, as it raised new and important issues for consideration. The NPSA is currently developing information for patients and a training program for nurses on infusion pumps.

2

The Patient's Role in Safety: A Physician's Perspective

Joel Mattison, M.D., FACS

The past half century has seen incredible changes in medicine as well as in the world at large. Recently, a "great awakening" seems to be entering medical ranks. Those of us in medicine are now more willing to learn from other disciplines and industries. There is less sensitivity about protecting our profession from public scrutiny and criticism. The very essence of medicine, the patient-doctor relationship, is undergoing considerable adjustment. Having practiced as a surgeon for many years, I have experienced all aspects of this transformation, and, like many physicians, I initially yearned for the good old days. Like anyone dealing with change, my understanding and acceptance of the revolution in medical practice was not a discrete, single event. I gradually moved from being uninterested (precontemplation stage) to considering the changes (contemplation stage) to deciding and preparing to adjust (action stage). These stages must be understood and heeded if we are to avoid becoming dinosaurs.

For the most part, the dominance of the medical model effectively suppressed the voice of the health care consumer. Paternalism was probably one of the most significant and yet subtle influences standing in the way of doctor-patient communication. And yet, like many in my profession, I saw no compelling need to relinquish the paternalistic role. In the early 1990s I wrote a review of a motion picture, *The Doctor,* for the *Journal of the American Medical Association.* This film was an adaptation of the book *A Taste of My Own Medicine,* by Dr. Edward E. Rosenbaum, originally published by Random House in 1988. In the book, Rosenbaum, a rheumatologist in Portland, Oregon, recounted his experiences undergoing treatment for cancer of the larynx. He wrote about his frustrations with the medical system, which included a delay in his diagnosis and a frequent display of indifference and lack of compassion by physicians and other caregivers. At the end of the 1991 movie version of this book, the physician (played by William Hurt) is both recovered and converted and in the last scene is requiring his residents to spend 72 hours as hospital patients as part of their medical training.

Needless to say, my review of Rosenbaum's book moved me further along toward the action stage in my professional transformation. It was hard not to appreciate the significance of the patient's point of view as recounted by Dr. Rosenbaum. About this same time the Picker/Commonwealth Program for Patient-Centered Care was established at Boston's Beth Israel Hospital and the Harvard Medical School. Initial research by this group culminated in the publication of the groundbreaking book *Through the Patient's Eyes* (Jossey-Bass Publishers, 1993). Not long after, the *Journal of the American Medical Association* regularly began to publish patient's stories in the "A Piece of My Mind" column, and similar patient testimonials were published in other medical journals. The era of patient-centered care was in full swing, and many physicians, including myself, were becoming convinced that the voice of the patient deserved greater attention. Studies of consumer attitudes supported this sentiment. In one such study, physician-patient communication was identified by 57 percent of American respondents as an essential indicator of quality.[1]

But does the patient have a role to play in reducing medical errors? There is proven value to involving patients in medical decision making, yet the merit of patient involvement in the safety movement may still be an enigma for many physicians. I doubt if a patient would be able to prevent an inadvertent intraoperative injury or notice that the surgical sponge count was inaccurate. Even in cases of a delayed diagnosis, it would be unlikely that a layperson could immediately recognize and correct the clinician's error.

When the issue of patient safety comes up, physicians commonly envision incidents attributable to inappropriate practitioner decisions or actions. I agree that the average patient wouldn't have sufficient knowledge or the ability to prevent such mistakes from being made. On the other hand, the medical profession has heard repeatedly over the past several years that errors most often result from a complex interplay of multiple factors and only rarely are due to the carelessness, perversity, or misconduct of single individuals. The patient is one of the players in this complex system of care, and yet we often think of patients in a passive way as the victims of errors and safety failures.

Patients can play an active part in preventing mistakes and ensuring their own safety if given the correct information and the right tools for the job. For example, when the doctor discusses common medication side effects with a patient, he or she is better prepared to recognize unexpected problems.

Described in the remainder of this chapter are approaches that physicians and other health care providers can use to involve patients actively in error prevention. Some of these suggestions originate from my professional experiences as a surgeon and my administrative work in clinical resource management at St. Joseph's Hospital of St. Joseph's–Baptist Health Care in Tampa, Florida. In addition, not long ago I had the opportunity as a patient to view the health care system from the patient's vantage point. This perspective made me realize the importance of strengthening the medical profession's resolve to collaborate with patients. It wasn't until I became a surgical patient that I fully realized the significance of the phrase "nothing about me, without me," apparently first voiced by an English midwife at a Salzburg seminar in 1988.[2]

Involving Patients in Safety

Patient participation in health care safety improvement must start with dialogue. The word *dialogue* comes from the Greek word *dialogos. Dia* means "through" and *logos* means "the word" or "the principle behind the spoken word." Dialogue is different from discussion. When two people or groups are dialoguing, the goal is collaboration with everyone involved coming out winners. In a discussion, each person or group is trying to convince the other of the correctness of an opinion or position. Simply put, effective dialogue can allow clinicians and patients to put aside the traditional dominance-subordination structure to achieve the common goal of safety.

It is important to use creative thinking and approaches that facilitate real two-way communication between providers and patients. Although certainly worthwhile, simply putting a patient or two on a health service advisory committee is clearly not sufficient to ensure meaningful dialogue. To improve the safety of health care services, we need to involve as many voices as possible, the pleasant (those who agree with us) and the not so pleasant (those who don't). Only by sharing all possible solutions to the safety problems in health care will substantial improvements be made. Physicians and other professionals must help patients understand what is needed from them in order to make the health care experience safer. Next, providers must find out what patients need to feel safe.

Helping Patients Understand Their Role

The long and often challenging process of sharing information and making it meaningful for patients has several aspects. Like many hospitals, St. Joseph's in Tampa distributes patient brochures to facilitate communication. Everyone entering as an inpatient is given a *Patient Information Guide* before leaving the admitting office. Included in the guide is a page entitled "10 Tips to Help Us Keep You Safe" (see figure 2-1). In addition to the "10 Tips," I would like to add some particular individualized examples of one-on-one suggestions that caregivers could offer hospitalized patients.

1. Make yourself easily and instantly recognizable and not just the patient in "B bed." Using a black "wide" felt tip pen, print your name in large letters on a thick (card stock) sheet of white paper that is at least $8^{1}/_{2} \times 11$ inches. Do not use longhand or ornamental styles in writing your name. Do

not add other information to the sign, even if you think it would be helpful to your caregivers. Tape or otherwise affix this sign to the head of your hospital bed or to the wall above the head of the bed. This sign provides one more way for caregivers to identify you.

Figure 2-1. Safety Suggestions in the Patient Information Guide at St. Joseph's Hospital, Tampa, Florida

10 Tips to Help Us Keep You Safe: Research has shown that the best way to prevent medical errors is for patients and families to take an active part in their medical care. You can play an important role by following these simple tips.

1. Make sure every health care team member who cares for you checks your name band. Please help us by keeping your identification bracelet in place until discharge.

2. Ask us any questions you may have. Discuss your concerns. Ask a family member or friend to speak for you if you are not able to speak for yourself.

3. Let us help you out of bed until we know you are steady on your feet. We do not want you to fall.

4. Give us complete and correct information about your health history, personal habits (such as alcohol use or smoking), and diet.

5. Make sure we know what medicine(s) you take. This includes what is ordered by a doctor and what you take on your own (such as aspirin or cold remedies). Include vitamins, herbs, and diet supplements.

6. Ask what each medicine is for. Learn about medicine side effects. Tell us if you think you are having a side effect.

7. Find out why a test or treatment is needed and how it may help you.

8. Ask your doctor about the results of your tests. Do not assume that "No news is good news."

9. Feel free to ask health care team members if they have washed their hands before they provide care to you. Good hand washing is still the best simple way to prevent the spread of germs.

10. Be sure you know what to expect when you go home and know what to report to your doctor.

Source: Publications Department, St. Joseph's Hospital, Tampa, Florida. Reprinted with permission.

2. If an anesthesiologist visits you prior to a surgery, tell him or her about any medications that you have been taking, even if you have stopped taking them. This is particularly important for medications containing steroids. Some effects of steroids continue for months after being discontinued. It is necessary for the anesthesiologist and any other treating physicians to know any history of steroid usage to avoid potential serious problems.

3. Some patients mistakenly assume that food allergies won't be a problem during the hospital stay. Although this seems to bear witness to a patient's trust in the system, it is important that the hospital caregivers are told about any food allergies. It is easier to avoid the problem than to treat it after it becomes full blown.

4. Everyone tends to forget things, and the stress of being a patient in the hospital may make the tendency even worse. Keep a small notepad and pencil at your bedside to jot down thoughts that might otherwise be lost during those temporary memory lapses.

Physicians must also share with patients the often difficult and sensitive issue of the potential for individual mistakes (for example, wrong-site surgery, diagnoses delays, incorrect medication prescriptions). We must help our patients to understand these potentials so that they may help us to guard against them.

What can a patient do to decrease the likelihood that practitioners will make a mistake? From the standpoint of reducing wrong-site surgeries, it is frequently valuable to give the patient a brochure describing the procedure (or even a general brochure on all procedures). In addition, proper informed consents and written operative permits can be effective safeguards if patients are encouraged to speak up with questions or concerns.

Reducing unnecessary risk exposure through the use of multiple safeguards can eliminate many errors, yet it is not always an easy thing to do. Ideally, each process has repeated checks to ensure that everything is proceeding correctly. For example, a nurse comes to the patient's hospital bedside with a pink pill. The patient asks, "Is this my heart medicine?" Nurse's answer, "Yes." Patient: "How do you know?" Nurse's answer: "I got it out of a labeled stock bottle." Patient persists, "How do you know that the bottle was labeled correctly and the drug was not past the expiration date?" (Etc.) We eventually come to some point in the process at which further checks would be absurd or at least not helpful (e.g., "How do you know that the source of this Digoxin was real Fox Glove?"). At such a point, we have to accept the source or else trust that the information we have is correct or at least adequate.

A similar interaction can transpire when the patient asks the clinician, "How do you know who I am?" or "How do I know who you are?" or "How do you know what is in the pill cup?" There is some point at which one has to settle for the best available information and depend on common sense. Knowing one from the other is a matter of judgment. Tina Long, an excellent nurse at St. Joseph's Hospital, once put it this way: "I think that we eventually just have to stop at some reasonable point and say, 'I believe that we have enough information to go ahead and give this medication.'" The human race is so interdependent that in some instances we can only move forward on the basis of well-founded trust.

When we think about inpatient safety, the subject of delirium (acute confusional state) in elderly hospitalized patients comes up only rarely. Delirium, however, is common and a serious source of morbidity and mortality among older hospitalized patients. If we are interested in safety, we can ill afford to ignore these facts. Delirium can be caused or aggravated by cognitive impairment, sleep deprivation, immobility, visual impairment, hearing impairment, and dehydration.[3] Primary prevention is probably the most effective treatment strategy. Despite our best efforts, however, confusion will still continue to be a problem for some patients. In these situations, the patient's family or friends should be actively recruited to serve as safety advocates on the patient's behalf. However, even young, relatively healthy patients may be unable to fully participate in error prevention activities. That may be why nearly half of the consumer participants in a recent unpublished study at St. Joseph's

Hospital said that it is best to have family or friends on hand to monitor care.

Seeking and Using Patient Feedback

It is not uncommon to find in the "Patient Rights and Responsibilities" statement given to hospitalized patients a sentence like "We will provide the best health care possible in a safe, clean, quiet, and pleasant environment." This promise is found under the heading of facility responsibilities, but there is usually no corollary statement listed in the patient rights section. Shouldn't we be telling patients that they have the right to feel safe while receiving care at the hospital? Perhaps that is what we think we are saying when we ask patients to answer questions completely so that clinicians can provide better care.

We probably cannot tell patients too often that health care team members use the identification bracelet on their wrist to confirm patient identity before medications are given or treatments initiated. Does cautioning patients to always call the nurse for help in getting out of bed help them feel safe? I would think so, but I can't say for sure. This brings us to the second component of effective dialogue: seeking feedback from patients and using it to create a safer environment.

Physicians and other health care professionals must avoid stereotyped thinking about what makes patients feel safe. When the dialogue is only one-sided, all we have is a discussion in which medical professionals try to convince patients to give us what we need to keep them safe. To turn this discussion into a dialogue, we have to discover from patients what they need from us to feel safe. Patients and medical professionals don't always have the same ideas about the relative importance of safety issues. These differences became apparent when St. Joseph's–Baptist Health Care started asking patients about their safety concerns.[4] The feedback commonly falls into the following six general categories:

1. *Universal precautions.* For example: Caregivers not washing hands, not wearing personal protective equipment, not following isolation protocols

2. *Sharps.* For example: Sharps containers overflowing, needles left in room from a previous patient, needle cap found in bed

3. *Medications.* For example: Nurses not washing hands, not checking patient's identification band prior to medication administration, not explaining the purpose for medications

4. *Shower/bath.* For example: Not clean, too much clutter, dirty bedside commode

5. *Cleanliness.* For example: Dirty bathroom, dirty patient room, dirty privacy curtains

6. *Slip/trip/fall/clutter.* For example: Too much clutter in halls and bathroom, uneven gravel on outdoor paths, uneven floor surfaces at door entryways

Many of these safety concerns are not the dramatic ones that most medical professionals would view as a high priority, yet this is what patients notice and tell us about in our questionnaire. Patients seem more focused on safety issues than on error issues (such as wrong-site surgery). This, of course, could be a very subtle and interesting form of denial. However, the survey results do heighten our awareness of what makes patients feel safe. Issues that draw the most attention from patients fall into the slip/trip/fall/clutter category. A preliminary goal for our hospital is to learn which categories of safety concerns receive the greatest number of comments from patients and then to resolve some of these concerns. In addition, the feedback has made us realize that patients need help in understanding the error aspects of safety that are worthy of *their* attention. The patient safety movement will not be complete if the patient perspective is not brought into the dialogue. The patient must be involved in many aspects of health care service that have an impact on safety, such as the following:

- Helping to reach an accurate diagnosis
- Deciding on appropriate treatment or management strategy
- Choosing a suitably experienced and safe provider (with current appropriate certification and verified training)

- Ensuring that treatment is appropriately administered, monitored, and adhered to
- Identifying side effects or adverse events quickly and taking appropriate action[5]

By dialoguing with patients, the flow of information can go in both directions. Ultimately this will have a positive impact on both safety and error-related concerns.

Improving Safety from the Ground Up

In any project, the greatest judgment is required in deciding how far back toward zero to take any existing system for which improvement is intended. This is true for the restoration of antiques and classic cars, almost any complex surgical case, and for any finely tuned business enterprise. How far back does one go in removing old paint, what is to be done with rusted or dented hardware, and how does one decide when or whether to replace or repair? If, in restoration, one removes too much of the real thing, it may be analogous to the collector who was perhaps overly proud of owning George Washington's original axe, adding that it had had two heads and five handles but was still completely original.

Trustee magazine recently carried an article about the $55 million replacement facility being built by St. Joseph's Community Hospital in West Bend, Wisconsin.[6] The new hospital building, which will be completed in May 2005, was designed for improved patient safety. "Spaces clearly have an impact on safety," said St. Joseph's Community Hospital CEO John Reiling. "We looked at the relationship between technology, equipment, and the physical plant and their impact on each other. How could we translate this information to design around patient safety?"

To answer this question, a "learning lab" was sponsored with the University of Minnesota's Carlson School of Management. In attendance were more than two dozen patient safety experts; local and national leaders in health care administration, research, and systems engineering; human behavior researchers; hospital quality improvement professionals; accreditation specialists; medical educators; hospital architects; nurses; pharmacists; and physicians. Hospital planners have traditionally decided on the physical layout first when designing a new building, but in the learning lab, participants learned how to *look at processes before deciding on space*— playing out how technology and structure could best assist those processes. In designing the new building, St. Joseph's Hospital in West Bend started with a list of the following top 10 priorities:

1. Failure analysis should be ongoing.
2. Stakeholder input is critical.
3. Accountable leadership is needed to drive the process.
4. Design should focus on organizational processes.
5. Design should reflect an understanding of human factors.
6. Design should occur with vulnerable populations in mind.
7. Design should be flexible enough to accommodate change.
8. Design should be standardized whenever possible.
9. Design should facilitate immediate access to information.
10. Design should address known threats to patient safety.

Unfortunately, few health care organizations are given the opportunity to start from scratch. It is often hard just to take the dramatic step of discarding some of the oldest of the old and embracing the affordable new. It is clear, however, that this new kind of thinking and planning is the wave of the future. For the present, many organizations will have to compromise somewhat and look for patient safety improvements wherever they can be achieved, even in small increments.

Engendering a Passion for Safety

Safety awareness is not communicated by rote or rules alone. Inspiration and example are a start, but these are only successful when safe habits have permeated our beings, etched our souls, and become second nature. For example, those of us in surgery cannot force ourselves to scratch our noses after we have scrubbed and gowned up. This is an unforgivable sin, and compliance was ingrained while our paint was still wet. We are also unable to cross that thin red line in an operating suite in street clothes. This is such a fervent religious conviction that it never comes to mind to question why. Whether something bad will happen is moot, because crossing the line is simply unthinkable.

Seeing clinicians compulsively stop to wash their hands before entering a patient's room spreads the idea that this safe practice is woven into our lives and that everyone is working to keep the environment clean. Changes in behavior and attitude come about, not through signs or repetition alone, but through teaching by example. Someone once asked Albert Schweitzer if example was the best way of teaching, to which he replied, "It is the only way." His hospital at Lambaréné, in western Gabon, was built on this principle, and his patients largely followed his example (and that of his staff). Many arguments on nearly all subjects at Lambaréné were settled with the reminder in Schweitzer's own words, "It is commanded that we not do that."[7] Hardly a day would pass without someone's repeating this to a patient, employee, or visitor, and I cannot recall anyone's ever disputing this simple statement.

Is your hospital "littered"? What patients see as litter may (to us) mean only some variant of untidiness, whereas to patients every damp spot represents a urine spill and is a symbol of carelessness and an ominous warning sign. The only way to combat littered hallways is by precept and example. Health care professionals must create the impression that it is a sacrilege either to drop trash or to pass it by when it is in one's path. Patients and staff who see senior staff stop to pick up trash get the idea that *everyone* is working to keep the environment clean and safe.

A special word about "wet litter," or spills, leaks, and puddles. In addition to the appearance of slovenliness, these are a constant source of falls for patients and staff alike. And one very small thing: cover the patient, especially during transit. However uncomfortable shivering in a cold hall may be and however embarrassing the humility of being exposed, from the patient's viewpoint it is probably the indignity of being uncovered in a hallway that is most disturbing. Of course, it is important to prevent injury to patients, but attention to their dignity is a means of communicating concern. Caring for the whole patient is an element of safety often underrated by medical professionals but highly valued by patients. Did you ever notice how litter-borne edentulous patients always draw the sheet up to cover their toothless mouths? These are only a few examples of the ways in which health care professionals can help patients to understand that we are a caring family in a safe facility. In many organizations, these behaviors and attitudes require a cultural change. Schweitzer's constant references to "reverence for life" were always evidence of his caring and respect for all living things.

Elaine Fantle Shimberg of Tampa, Florida, has written some 16 helpful books for patients. She usually works with a medical expert, and her information is understandable, well organized, and trustworthy. One of her best books, coauthored with Dr. Sheldon Blau, is *How to Get Out of the Hospital Alive* (Macmillian, 1997). This is not necessarily a book you'd want to give to an anxious friend who is just now entering the hospital for surgery. But it is certainly a book that will be an indispensable complement to your medical knowledge as you learn how patients think and react at a very vulnerable time. Read it with an open mind; it is filled with truths that physicians altogether too often think are beneath their notice.

Encouraging Provider-Patient Dialogue

Leading patients to see the importance of their attention to, and understanding of, their contribution to safety is a relatively new challenge for the medical profession. We must learn what seems most important to patients if we seriously covet their cooperation in eliminating or minimizing the potential for error. The principles of teaching by example are probably always the best solution to this problem. The medical professional must genuinely solicit patient opinions and seek patients' informed cooperation. As we come to learn, understand, and accept more of the theories of error, and as we learn how to share this information with our patients, we can look forward to safer days and safer environments for all of us. All health care professionals must remain open and inquisitive about the viewpoints of those for whom it is our special privilege to care in a time of need.

Consumer involvement in the patient safety movement is an imperative. The public and our patients need to understand the risk in health services and participate with us in reducing that risk. At times this means forming partnerships with other physicians or nurses, for example, in improving medication safety and avoiding wrong-site surgery. At other times it means becoming educated consumers and realizing that there may be trade-offs between patient comfort and increased risk, as in the case of conscious sedation.

Patient safety will not be improved until everyone acknowledges that risks exist at all levels of health care. A safer way of caring for patients can be achieved by detecting, measuring, and monitoring risk, accompanied by steadfast determination. Safety is a continually evolving property of a complex system, especially a system as complex as modern medical care. It is a certainty that the sources of harm will change as medical care changes. Safety will be a never-ending, but important, aspect of the medical professional's work. The good news is that it can be one of those true "win-win-win" situations for our patients, for all of us who deliver health care, and for our provider institutions.

What a lot of sick compulsivity and extra effort we're talking about here! Keep in mind, however, that safety is the end result of unbridled altruism and never-fading enthusiasm. But if that is not reason enough, remember that you are a part of designing medical safety policy that may some day be a matter of life or death to you or your family. As a card-carrying member of society, remember that the life you save by some degree of excessive compulsivity may be your own. Is this too much trouble? I doubt it. The elevator is here and waiting at the bottom floor. Join in, and let's go up together.

References

1. *National Survey on Americans as Health Care Consumers: An Update on the Role of Quality Information.* Kaiser Family Foundation/Agency for Healthcare Research and Quality (Menlo Park, Calif: Henry J. Kaiser Family Foundation, 2000).
2. *National Agenda for Action: Patients and Families in Patient Safety* (Chicago: The National Patient Safety Foundation, 2003).
3. S. K. Inouye and others, "A Multicomponent Intervention to Prevent Delirium in Hospitalized Older Patients," *New England Journal of Medicine* 340, no. 9 (1999): 669–76.
4. There are a total of 910 inpatient beds in the St. Joseph's–Baptist system (St. Joseph's Emergency Center, South Florida Baptist Hospital, St. Joseph's Hospital, St. Joseph's Children's Hospital, and St. Joseph's Women's Hospital).
5. C. A. Vincent and A. Coulter, "Patient Safety: What about the Patient?" *Quality and Safety in Health Care* 11 (2002): 76–80.
6. L. Larson, "Putting Safety in the Blueprint," *Trustee* 56, no. 2 (2003): 9–13.
7. J. Mattison, "Lessons from Lambarene, Part I," *Bulletin of the American College of Surgeons* 77, no. 9 (1999): 10–21.

3

Creating Opportunities for Patient Involvement in Error Prevention

Paula S. Swain, R.N., M.S.N., CPHQ, FNAHQ, and Patrice L. Spath, B.A., RHIT

A father is observed racing down a hospital hallway while talking on a cell phone. His anxiety is obvious as he advises the listener, "Do not let them give the baby anything until you see the vial that the medicine comes in."

This is an example of the consumer's fear response to media reports of unsafe health care situations. Alerts abound advising consumers of how to conduct themselves if they want to live to tell about their health care experience. The worst-case scenarios seem to surface to the top with the public's hearing about the dangers of hospital-acquired infections, medication mix-ups, significant physical injuries, and unfortunate equipment failures. On any given day we read news stories of errors in blood and donor typing, surgical removal of the wrong body parts, instruments and sponges left behind following operative procedures, and every type of medication error imaginable. Besides the tales of misadventure in the news media, a number of publicly available books describe the inner workings of health care. In one such book, *Complications,* physician-author Atul Gawande notes that whereas the public may think medicine is an orderly field of knowledge and procedure, it definitely is not. Gawande describes medicine as an imperfect science with constantly changing knowledge, uncertain information, and fallible individuals.[1]

Contrary to what the public may think, safety has always been a priority in health care. A number of safeguards, precautions, and process improvements are making health care delivery safer every day. Remarkably, only in the past few years has the patient safety movement encouraged the active involvement of patients. Patients were often viewed as the victims of errors and safety failures, but there is growing evidence that they have a role in *promoting safety*. When patients ask questions about their medications or an anticipated procedure, they are serving as safeguards in the system—a reminder to caregivers to recheck or validate that the right thing is being done.

Adding the patient to the health care system of checks and balances can help prevent what may have been a simple mistake from becoming a harmful error that reaches the patient. To gain the value of this additional safeguard, health care professionals must encourage patients to pay attention to the care being provided to them and speak up if something doesn't seem right. The act of clarification can serve as a "pause" in what might otherwise be a very complex or tightly coupled, high-risk process. A tightly coupled process is one in which the steps follow one another so closely that an error in one step cannot be recognized and responded to before the next step is well under way.[2]

Patients who know what to expect from the health care experience can check on the appropriate performance of clinical tasks. For example, practitioners should discuss the common side effects of a medication when prescribing something new for a patient. If such a discussion fails to occur, patients are ill prepared to cope with side effects and may not recognize unexpected problems. Failure to receive information about the side effects of a medication should prompt the patient to ask questions of the physician or pharmacist.

The health care industry is endorsing an active role for consumers in helping to reduce errors by encouraging patients to ask questions and be vigilant. For example, in September 2000, the American Hospital Association issued a Quality Advisory to its members urging them to improve medication safety by partnering with patients.[3] Health care providers were asked to take the lead in helping patients and other consumers learn as much as possible about safe medication use. In March 2002, the Joint Commission on Accreditation of Healthcare Organizations, together with the

Centers for Medicare and Medicaid Services, launched a national program to urge patients to take a role in preventing health care errors by becoming active, involved, and informed participants on the health care team.[4]

One of the goals of the National Patient Safety Foundation (NPSF) is to educate consumers on how they can become active partners with their health care team and help make sure they have a safer experience with the health care system. In support of this goal, the NPSF partnered with groups like the American Hospital Association and the American Medical Association to create brochures and fact sheets on such topics as "Preventing Infections in the Hospital—What You as a Patient Can Do."[5]

The National Council on Patient Information and Education, a coalition of nearly 200 organizations committed to safer, more effective medicine use, is seeking to improve the safety of medication use through increased consumer involvement.[6] In 2003, the council and the Agency for Healthcare Research and Quality jointly released a new resource called *Your Medicine: Play It Safe* to help consumers use prescription medicines safely.[7] These are just a few of the many initiatives that are being sponsored by different segments of the health care industry.

To effectively engage patients as active partners in the patient safety movement, health care professionals must first understand how things look from the patient's perspective. Patients want to be treated like responsible adults capable of assimilating information, asking informed questions, and having reasonable expectations. Yet the health care experience often falls short of these expectations. Consider how one patient described her recent stay at a large urban hospital for treatment of sepsis.

It was late, about 11:45 PM, on the first night of my hospital admission. I'd been in the hospital for 14 hours. My last recorded temperature was 103.2°F, and the first dose of antibiotic was just hung. The air in the room was still. The air-conditioning must have been off on this end of the hall. My husband was dozing in a chair by the bed. It is so hot that I can't breathe. My head is pounding and every inch of my body hurts.

I'm sure I will be left on my own tonight. At change of shift, the night nurse walked in and I requested "something" for my temperature and aching body, and air-conditioning. No one got back to me, so after an hour of waiting I used the call bell. "They" could not understand my request over the intercom and promised to come to my room. When the nurse stopped by and heard my request, she answered that she was pretty sure I had nothing ordered but would check. I suggested she call the physician for an order before it got too much later. Her body language told me I was on my own. I never saw her again.

I woke my husband and instructed him to get two rubber gloves from the box of rubber gloves in my room and go down to the nutrition room and fill each glove with ice. He was worried someone would confront him—I assured him no one would bother him at this late hour. Soon he came back with the gloves filled with ice. He quickly got the gist of cooling me and supplied me with towels to catch the melting ice dripping from my body. He found a basin and went back to the nutrition room and stocked up on more icy gloves.

Clearly, I "knew" too much, asked too many questions, was not the priority or whatever else was in the equation. I truly felt retaliated against and vowed I would do what I could on my own so I would not be sabotaged in my pursuit of health.

The patient, a registered nurse with previous bedside experience at another hospital, was forced by her illness to make the transition from caring for patients to being a patient herself. She found the stark realities of health care terrifying when viewed from the patient's vantage point. Her health care background would qualify her as an "activated patient"—a concept that emerged from work that has been done around the role of the patient in the so-called chronic disease model.[8] Activated patients are considered sufficiently informed and motivated to handle the day-to-day management of their chronic condition. Similar characteristics—informed and motivated—will help patients to be more effective partners in the patient safety movement. Yet as the patient's story of her hospitalization unfolds in this chapter, it will become apparent that the attitudes and actions of health care professionals must change if the goal of patient- and family-centered patient safety is to be realized.

New Attitudes and Actions

Health care providers now have access to a large array of patient safety materials that can be shared with patients. However, these materials will not meet the intended goal of consumer involvement in patient safety until practitioners and the health care system embrace patients as valuable and active partners. First and foremost, health care professionals must truly believe that patients have an important role in reducing mistakes in the delivery of health care services. The need to include patients in the process of care was one of the safety improvement principles advanced in the Institute of Medicine's 1999 report *To Err Is Human: Building a Safer Health System.*[9] In support of this principle, numerous medical professional groups, such as the American College of Physicians, have issued position statements describing the importance of involving patients in discussions and in the decision process.[10] Health care provider groups, such as The Minnesota Alliance for Patient Safety, have created brochures to explain to patients how they can make the health care experience safer.[11] The National Patient Safety Foundation is urging all hospitals, health systems, and national and local health care organizations to involve patients and families in systems and patient safety programs.[12]

The success of efforts to partner with patients and families for the purpose of improving safety will actually depend largely on the attitudes and actions of individual caregivers. It is fairly easy to embrace the concept of open and honest communication with patients to gain the information needed for diagnosis or treatment purposes. But what if those same patients question why the caregiver touched them without washing his or her hands first? Or question the need for a particular procedure? Will health care professionals be as accepting of collaboration when patients are challenging clinical practices or professional decisions? No one likes to have his or her judgment questioned, and the usual emotional response is to become defensive and angry. Consider how caregivers responded to questions asked by the patient hospitalized for treatment of sepsis.

I was told that I needed an infusion of a potent antibiotic to stop the sepsis that was forming in my body. However, because my peripheral veins were inadequate, I would need to have a percutaneous intravenous catheter (PIC line) inserted. The health care provider who installed the PIC line told me who should draw blood out of the catheter as well as how to manage the catheter before and after every antibiotic infusion. He also told me that this was the only access available to infuse the antibiotic, short of a more invasive procedure.

I felt responsible for assisting in maintaining the PIC line over the course of my treatment, which would take two weeks. I asked each new nurse that arrived to administer a dose of antibiotics if she or he had experience managing a PIC line. Another time I questioned a radiology technician who was planning to infuse contrast through the PIC line for a CT scan that had been ordered. When I asked questions, merely in an attempt to protect the PIC line, much of the time I was met with hostility and frustration by caregivers who reported that they were "just trying to do their jobs."

I got inconsistent messages from my caregivers and was worried about protecting the catheter. Thankfully, a thoughtful charge nurse finally put written instructions on how to maintain the PIC line on the door to my hospital room. This was after I'd taught 14 different nurses how to manage that line. I don't know if the radiology technician learned anything from our exchange, but I ended up having a CT scan without any contrast agent.

Professional attitudes influence actions. Most patients are keen to take responsibility for playing their part in trying to optimize treatment outcomes; however, many are frustrated by the lack of caregiver support in allowing them to satisfactorily fulfill this role.[13] Health care professionals may feel confronted and become defensive when the patient asks a question. In this situation, patients can easily become concerned about the safety of the care they are receiving. Physicians, nurses, and other health care professionals must learn how to interact and support patients who question their care. An ancient Buddhist story illustrates the type of communication gap that may exist between patients and health care professionals:

> The King said: "Venerable Nagasena, will you converse with me?" Nagasena: "If your majesty will speak with me as wise men converse, I will; but if your majesty converses with me as kings converse, I will not." "How then converse with the wise, venerable Nagasena?" "The wise do not get angry when they are driven into a corner; kings do."[14]

In a patient-safe culture, health care professionals must converse like wise men, not kings, when responding to inquisitive patients and/or family members. Caregivers may need coaching as well as education to narrow the communication gap. No patient should be afraid to ask a question, and no practitioner should appear offended by a patient who is willing to speak up. It helps to understand that patients may set high expectations or ask frequent questions in response to their own feelings of being out of control. It is the health care professional's job to facilitate a process whereby patients can regain control by validating patients' concerns, providing reassurance, and finding legitimate ways for patients to be actively involved. Caregivers must also be clear on the expectation that patients should inquire whenever they believe that care is not being provided in a safe manner. Consider how staff responses to the septic patient varied immediately after admission to the hospital.

My physician had urged me to hurry in getting to the hospital so that treatment would get started right away for the infection in my leg. Transportation from admissions to my hospital room seemed efficient enough. Yet once I got to my room, I was left alone. It soon became apparent there were other issues being dealt with on the floor that were more important than the "new admission in 624"!

During the first three hours, a few of the various staff members looked into my room. I couldn't get even an aspirin out of the group. No physician orders had come in, and the staff members appeared willing to wait until orders were called in. I wondered why no one had the initiative to call my physician? The obvious conclusion: "The staff don't care." Shift change added to the confusion. I asked for the nurse caring for me, but no one would commit. Finally, I asked to fill out my own assessment form and start the plan of care. After that, a nurse described as an "admitting nurse" sat down to take my health history. We bonded. Even though she knew nothing of my physician's orders, she listened to me, observed my wound, and heard my anxiety.

Effective Communication

One way to better understand how to communicate with patients would be to revitalize bedside teaching in medical schools. For a number of reasons, actual teaching at the bedside has declined from an incidence of 75 percent in the 1960s to an incidence of less than 16 percent in 1997.[15] Bedside teaching in medical schools, as in other settings of learning, is very well suited for using role modeling as a technique for teaching patient collaboration strategies. Although it is possible to describe appropriate communication skills, it is far more effective to demonstrate those skills through interactions with actual patients. Adults attach more meaning to learning gained from actual experience than that gained from passive learning.[16] And several studies have shown that a majority of patients enjoy the bedside teaching experience and feel that it helps them better understand their conditions.[17]

Some of the principles and benefits of the bedside teaching experience are evident in the collaborative practice models of patient care that hospitals and other health care providers are implementing. For example, "interdisciplinary rounding" is a component of the collaborative care model in the cardiac surgery unit at Concord Hospital in Concord, New Hampshire.[18] Members of the cardiac care team come together at one time each day to make rounds at each patient's bedside. Family members are encouraged to be present, and the patient and family members are encouraged to participate in the rounds process. Every effort is made to speak in ordinary language instead of medical terminology. In addition to discussing the patient's progress and treatment plan, the patient, family members, and cardiac care team members are asked about anything that didn't go as expected, or "system glitches." Ever since the morning rounds process was implemented, patients and family members have reported knowing exactly what is happening and what is planned. At first, practitioners felt uncomfortable discussing clinical situations openly with patients and family members and accepting their input. With time, however, participants became more at ease, and now practitioners frequently comment about how rewarding the rounds process is and how much it means to patients and families.

Health care professional groups are developing hands-on training resources to teach their members the communication skills that are important in creating an understanding and trusting relationship with patients. The American Academy of Orthopaedic Surgeons (AAOS) was one of the first medical associations to offer such training. The AAOS communication skills mentoring program, developed in collaboration with the Bayer Institute for Health Care Communication in West Haven, Connecticut,[19] was initiated in 2001 after AAOS public opinion surveys revealed that the American public view orthopedic surgeons as "high tech, low touch."[20] These half-day communication skills workshops are very interactive, with only 20 percent of the time spent on didactic teaching. Orthopedic-specific video vignettes of medical interviews combined with role-playing, discussions, and feedback make up the majority of the workshop.[21]

John R. Tongue, M.D., a practicing orthopedic surgeon in Tualatin, Oregon, and chair of the AAOS Communications Skills Project Team, has published an online list of patient interview tips that are based on his interviews with over 100,000 orthopedic patients as well as on the Bayer Institute's "Clinician-Patient Communication Course."[22] The AAOS has also pioneered the "Sign

Your Site" program to reduce wrong-site surgical errors. Dr. Tongue has adapted the academy's recommendations as follows:

In my practice my nurse, Jessie, simply tells every patient during the preoperative visit that I will be marking his or her surgery site. Then I mark the incision site itself and say, "I'll mark this more carefully in surgery." I place my initials on the patient's arm or leg. I think patients must feel a little strange being marked, so I sometimes say, "This is so they don't put you in the wrong room and take your gall bladder out!" They seem to really enjoy the comment, sometimes laughing loudly. Occasionally, if the patient seems nervous before my signing/marking, I'll say, "You know, there were a few famous orthopedic surgeons who didn't make it through their 30-year careers keeping left and right straight! So I need to do this in my practice." Humility wins them over. My mark is made the day before the surgery, so I also reassure them that the mark will still be there after washing. And I look at all marks in the preop holding area immediately before surgery. I prefer to sign/mark in my office in advance as a way of educating the patient in a less stressful environment, but that won't work in all practice settings.

Patient can mark "yes" over my marks or "no" on the opposite side that won't be operated on. This does even more to assure them and the reviewing surgical team that we're all on the same page. Some patients might feel it isn't necessary to repeat the process, whereas others may think it's great (reassuring) to reconfirm the site.[23]

Active Listening

The ability to communicate effectively is vital to the practitioner-patient partnership. And how the practitioner says something can be even more important than what is actually said. The spoken words are important, but they aren't the only way in which messages are conveyed. It is estimated that as much as 93 percent of communication includes such nonverbal behaviors as tone of voice, mannerisms, and body language.[24] Caregivers who are proficient in active listening skills can greatly enhance the provider-patient relationship, as evidenced by the experiences of the patient mentioned earlier who was hospitalized for treatment of sepsis.

Was the care I was receiving safe? My perceptions were influenced by staff member reactions to my questions and suggestions. Some technicians took the time to listen to me as I described the best site for a phlebotomy or how to position me so that my leg wound would be protected. I felt these staff members not only respected me, but they also cared about my safety.

Listening effectively is hearing and understanding what the other person is saying. Health care providers must learn to be empathetic listeners, especially when the patient or family member is expressing a quality or safety concern. Chances are that many health care professionals have instinctively, or through practice, developed the skill of empathy; empathetic listening thus appears to be the easiest patient collaboration tool to learn. Yet this skill is often neglected in the hectic day-to-day delivery of health care services. And this oversight widens the gap between providers and patients, creating even greater safety concerns.

A University of Maine researcher, Dr. Marisue Pickering, identified four characteristics of empathetic listeners as follows:

1. Desire to be other-directed rather than to project one's own feelings and ideas onto the other

2. Desire to be nondefensive rather than to protect the self. When the self is being protected, it is difficult to focus on another person.

3. Desire to imagine the roles, perspectives, or experiences of the other rather than assuming they are the same as one's own

4. Desire to listen as a receiver, not as a critic, and desire to understand the other person rather than to achieve either agreement from, or change in, that person[25]

Some health care organizations are offering training sessions to help caregivers be more open and empathetic with patients. Skills taught in these training sessions include the following:

- Use of verbal and nonverbal communication to acknowledge input or questions from patients
- How to respond to the patient's verbal message through restating or paraphrasing
- Use of cues to reflect the patient's feelings, experiences, or statements
- How to offer tentative interpretations that reflect the patient's feelings, desires, or meanings
- Use of summarizing or synthesizing strategies to focus the feelings and/or concerns of patients
- How to respond when the patient requests more information or expresses confusion about some aspect of the health care experience
- How to support patients and families by showing warmth and caring
- How to check perceptions in a nondefensive manner to find out if the patient's interpretations and perceptions are valid and accurate
- How to give patients time to think as well as talk

George Bernard Shaw once wrote, "The greatest problem with communication is the illusion that it has been accomplished." Communication is an essential part of the social contract between practitioners and patients. So, when a patient and provider come together, building communication and collaboration can reduce poor outcomes and improve the patient's safety. As health care professionals come to appreciate the value and expertise of patients and families in reducing adverse events, the role of better communication will be evident. Communication is not just saying words; it is creating true understanding between caregivers and patients. Active listening is an important skill in that process.

Building Organizational Commitment

The organization acts as a host to the health care team, and as such, the manner in which the organization carries out the business of health service markedly affects the actions and attitudes of care-givers. Senior leaders determine overall purpose and policies and are responsible for decisions about how policies apply to physicians, nurses, and other members of the patient care team. The importance of partnering with patients and families to improve safety must be legitimized within the broader organization. A patient-centered culture of patient safety cannot be mandated administratively nor can it be philosophically idealized into existence. Removing the division between patients and families on the one hand and providers on the other requires a fundamental shift in the culture of the organization. And culture change starts at the top.

Models for Culture Change

Experiences in changing the culture of safety at the Dana-Farber Cancer Institute (DFCI) in Boston, Massachusetts, have become a model for other organizations seeking to build better partnerships with patients and families. At DFCI, patients and families are treated as partners in care design, delivery, assessment, and improvement. Patients participate in the following arenas:

- Adult and pediatric patient and family advisory committees
- The adult oncology clinical services committee, during which discussion includes errors, falls, and other patient safety issues
- Facility planning
- Patient care rounds
- The patient educator program (cancer patients teach medical fellows about being a patient)
- The complementary therapy task force
- Friday meetings with the administrator[26]

Children's Hospital and Clinics in Minneapolis is another organization committed to involving patients and families in the health care experience. In 1999 the board of directors adopted quality and safety as an ethical obligation and the organization's number-one shared value.[27] Through focused discussions with family members, the organization's senior leaders discovered what families already knew—patient care is risky and errors do occur. Families were looking for ways to be involved in safety improvement, and because the organization saw this as an opportunity to partner with patients and their families, it adopted a policy of open and honest communication with patients and families. The time, place, and circumstances of medical errors, as well as the consequences and actions taken to treat or ameliorate them, are shared. Senior leaders agreed that however bad the truth is, only one thing could be worse: never telling the truth and eliminating the opportunity for something to be done to prevent the mistake from happening again.

Julianne Morath, chief operating officer at Children's Hospitals and Clinics of Minneapolis and 2002 winner of the John Eisenberg Award for Lifetime Achievement in Patient Safety, emphasizes that improved safety requires a partnership among members of the health care team and the patient and family members. In fact, says Morath, a culture of partnership is one of four important aspects of a safety culture. The other three aspects are an accountable culture, a just culture, and a culture of continuous learning.[28]

Patient and family partnerships are an important element in an organization's patient safety initiative. This component is clearly evident in the work being done at Murray-Calloway County Hospital in Murray, Kentucky. There is a clear top-down commitment to patient safety improvement (see figure 3-1). This commitment is articulated in many ways, such as the following:

- Multidisciplinary patient-resident safety committee, which includes physicians
- Patient safety integrated into the "Leadership Plan for Provision of Patient Care"
- Routine reporting from the patient-resident safety committee to the organization's leaders through the medical executive committee, quality council, and the governing board,

using a "Performance Improvement Priority Dashboard" of patient safety issues

- Organizational shift in philosophy from punitive to "no blame" through implementation of the following:

    —Anonymous reporting option for medication errors (Staff members who self-report receive a thank-you note expressing appreciation for the employee's commitment to safety and for upholding the organization's value of honesty.)

Figure 3-1.   Organizational Safety Triangle at Murray-Calloway County Hospital

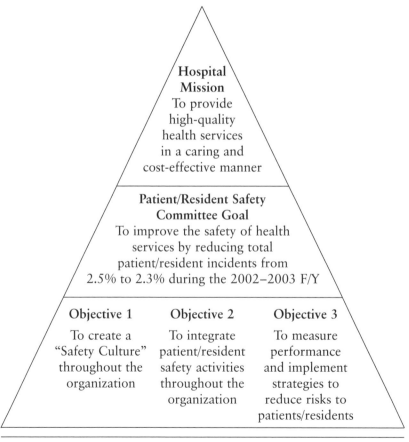

Hospital
Mission
To provide
high-quality
health services
in a caring and
cost-effective manner

**Patient/Resident Safety
Committee Goal**
To improve the safety of health
services by reducing total
patient/resident incidents from
2.5% to 2.3% during the 2002–2003 F/Y

Objective 1

To create a
"Safety Culture"
throughout the
organization

Objective 2

To integrate
patient/resident
safety activities
throughout the
organization

Objective 3

To measure
performance
and implement
strategies to
reduce risks to
patients/residents

Source: Murray-Calloway County Hospital, Patient/Resident Safety Committee Goals and Objectives, 2002–2003. Reprinted with permission from Murray-Calloway County Hospital, Murray, Kentucky.

—A copy of the note goes to the staff's director, who later uses the information as a positive element in the annual performance evaluation.

- Staff attendance required at patient safety–related training, including creation of a safety-conscious culture and patient partnership techniques
- Patient education provided through participation in a "Speak Up" campaign that covers all of the organization's entities: hospital, nursing home, home care, and hospice
- Staff participation in defining the "ABCs of Patient-Resident Safety" in the unique areas of the organization

Demonstrating Commitment to the Patient

Nationwide attention is focused on the creation of health care provider "report cards" that allow consumers to make informed choices when selecting providers. Whether public access to comparative data on quality and outcomes will significantly impact consumer choice has yet to be determined. However, heightened media attention on patient safety has sensitized consumers to the realization that things can go wrong during the delivery of health care services.

Can a patient or family member determine whether a health care organization is truly committed to patient safety? The answer may not be apparent in a public report card about that organization's performance, but consumers most likely form an opinion about the safety of an organization through personal experiences and/or reports from those who have had personal experiences.[29] Even though patients and their families may be uninformed in matters of technical or clinical performance, they are often able to discern an organization's commitment to safety through the attitudes and actions of caregivers. The experiences of the patient who was hospitalized for treatment of sepsis illustrate the consumer's perspective.

The view from the bedside is a trusting position until expectations run amuck. The patient's capacity to hear all the discussion over many shifts creates a sense of inconsistency. There is fear that a thin thread is holding the treatment together, and perhaps the unthinkable will happen and the patient will become a victim.

As time passes in my hospital stay, a familiar routine emerges. Running the antibiotic through the line takes one hour. The antibiotic drip needs to start by a certain time so that other treatments, such as my trip to physical therapy, can be under way by 10 in the morning. This sounds simple, but inefficiencies and the possibility of breaking the thread of safety abound.

What if the antibiotic is started just half an hour late? The treatment might not be finished by the time I go to the physical therapy department for a whirlpool treatment on my leg wound. The facility has only one whirlpool, lots of people in the hospital need treatments, and the physical therapy department has a tight schedule. What if I miss my scheduled whirlpool treatment time because the antibiotic hasn't finished infusing? Or if I go to physical therapy with the IV still running, will a nurse leave the floor and find me to flush the line when the antibiotic has finished running in? I was told that flushing the line is important; otherwise, I might lose critical access. Then what?

Issues that seemed inconsequential to me when I was the bedside nurse have taken on a whole different meaning now that I am a patient. When I share my fears with staff members, they seem to brush me off. One of the wheels on the IV pole is broken and won't swivel and is why I need a nurse to help me go to the bathroom when the IV is running in. It takes an average of 14 1/2 minutes for a nurse to answer my call light. My bladder seldom lasts that long. I wonder if other, more important aspects of my treatment will go any better?

Organizations committed to patient safety do more than hand out pamphlets to inform patients that "It's okay to ask questions and to expect answers you understand." Personal safety is a common concern for all patients, yet for a variety of reasons many don't speak up when they are fearful of staff's making a mistake. That's why organizations committed to patient safety are proactive in partnering with patients and family members. Everyone must be willing to admit that mistakes can happen and be upfront in explaining to patients what is being done to reduce the chance of errors (including what the patient can do). The more often that patients can be made to feel in control of a seemingly out-of-control situation, the greater their sense of safety and camaraderie with the health care team. As patients' feelings of control rise, so will their willingness to speak up when something doesn't seem to be going just right.

Empowering Patients with Information

Whose responsibility is it to educate patients about their role in patient safety? Since the 1999 release of the Institute of Medicine's report *To Err Is Human: Building a Safer Health System,* a number of national and state governmental agencies and organizations have undertaken initiatives aimed at educating consumers about their role in preventing medical errors. "Be Involved in Your Health Care: Tips to Help Prevent Medical Errors," published by the Virginians Improving Patient Care and Safety in Richmond, Virginia, is just one of the many pamphlets and fact sheets that have been created at the state level to enlighten consumers.[30] Nationally, groups such as the Agency for Healthcare Research and Quality[31] and the Institute for Safe Medication Practices[32] have published numerous resources on what consumers can do to reduce medication errors and prevent untoward outcomes.

A component of the National Patient Safety Foundation's (NPSF's) Agenda for Action, "Nothing About Me, Without Me," includes the development and distribution of materials designed to arm consumers with the knowledge necessary to become active participants in the patient safety movement. To date, the NPSF has produced several safety publications for patients and families, including "Safety as You Go from Hospital to Home."[33] In March 2002 the NPSF Patient and Family Advisory Council launched a nationwide campaign, Patient Safety Awareness Week, to promote patients' involvement in their own care.[34] The Joint Commission on Accreditation of Healthcare Organizations has made its "Speak Up" brochures available to the public as well as to health care organizations.[35]

Consumer groups are also very much involved in getting the word out. For example, PULSE America is a not-for-profit organization working to reduce the rate of medical errors by educating the public and advocating a safer health care system.[36] The acronym PULSE stands for Persons United Limiting Substandards and Errors in Health Care. The not-for-profit group Parents of Infants and Children with Kernicterus has worked to educate health care professionals and the public about the dangers of severe newborn jaundice with the goal of preventing kernicterus, a condition that causes severe cerebral palsy.[37]

Patients as Safety Partners

The patient safety educational strategies for consumers are reminiscent of the initiatives undertaken in the early 1990s to familiarize the public with clinical practice guidelines. Developers of these guidelines created consumer-friendly versions for distribution to the public, and various groups incorporated guideline recommendations into patient teaching materials. Creating informed patients was considered an important strategy for improving practitioner compliance with the guidelines and reducing unnecessary costs associated with inappropriate care.[38] This strategy of creating informed patients continues today, with numerous mass information campaigns and consumer-directed education opportunities sponsored by payers, health care providers, and consumer groups. Now, more than 10 years after the concept of empowering patients with information was first introduced on a national level, many consumers have become informed and proactive in health care decision making.

The empowerment of patients to become partners in the patient safety movement is a logical extension of the consumer education initiatives started in the 1990s. Lessons learned during the earlier guideline education campaigns should be applied to the safety movement. One important feature of successful public education strategies is diversity. Education can be:

- Informal or formal
- Impersonal or personal
- One-way or interactive
- Isolated or connected to ongoing relationships
- Knowledge oriented or change oriented[39]

Already a number of practices and resources are aimed at encouraging patients to share responsibility for their own safety.[40] Although these initiatives are valuable, getting the message to individual consumers will require one-on-one interactions with health care providers. Research on the impact of different physician education strategies for implementing guidelines have indicated that personal, interactive strategies tended to be more influential in changing practitioner behavior than have more formal or indirect approaches.[41] This is an important lesson for those seeking to empower consumers with the knowledge to become more involved in health care safety.

The economist Joseph Schumpeter wrote in 1939 that "it was not enough to produce satisfactory soap, it was also necessary to induce people to wash." This sentiment was echoed by John Williamson in a 1991 contribution to a book from the American College of Physician Executives. Here Williamson emphasized that physicians needed to be educated on the importance of providing better information to patients about various treatment options and expected outcomes.[42] Similar practitioner education must occur as it relates to patient safety information.

Every contact between caregivers and consumers must be seen as an opportunity to disseminate information about the patient's role in safety. Physicians, nurses, and other caregivers must personally interact with patients and family members to impart information. Mass education campaigns will only be successful if the message is consistently reinforced at the patient-caregiver level. Some health care organizations have already begun to initiate one-on-one patient safety dialogues between caregivers and patients. Some examples of these efforts follow.

Partnership Initiatives That Work

Partnering with patients is a vital component of patient safety at Lovelace Health System in New Mexico. During the first phase of enacting a comprehensive patient safety program, education was provided to staff members on their responsibilities for patient safety and incident-reporting requirements. Once the various cultural barriers to an effective program were addressed, the organization was ready to move on to the next stage. The organization refers to this second step as the patient-focused, or "active," phase of patient safety. In this phase, caregivers actively partner with patients and families to reduce errors. This is done through a variety of techniques.

A hospitality coordinator visits each patient on admission. In addition to explaining the hospital routine, the coordinator gives the patient a "Tips for Safe Health Care" card (figure 3-2). The card contains the organization's patient safety slogan, "Together Improving Patient Safety," along with suggestions on how the patient can actively participate in his or her care and help ensure a safe health care experience. The card also contains the phone number of the organization's patient safety hotline, which patients and family members are urged to call if they have safety ideas, suggestions, or concerns. The organization's patient safety slogan and hotline number are also printed on a card included in the patient services guide, which is given to every patient at the time of admission (figure 3-3).

One clinic in the Lovelace Health System participates in a patient safety project sponsored by the American Medical Group Association and is entitled "Safety Collaborative for the Outpatient Environment." The project's goal is to decrease potentially harmful medication interactions, including prescription and over-the-counter medicines as well as herbal remedies. The project includes the following activities:

- Patients are contacted by telephone to remind them to bring to their next clinic appointment the medications they are taking or a list of those medications.

- During the patient's clinic visit, the nurse helps the patient complete a medication card that lists all medications the patient is taking and any allergies the patient may have.

- The nurse assesses the patient's medications to determine the potential for adverse drug reactions using Internet resources and/or pharmacy consultation.

Figure 3-2.   Lovelace Health System Patient Safety Program Tips for Safe Health Care

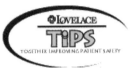 **Patient Safety Program Tips for Safe Health Care**

Your medical and personal safety is always a primary concern at Lovelace.

By actively participating with your health care team and following these patient safety guidelines, you can ensure a safe health care experience.

- **Speak up if you have questions or concerns.** You have the right to know about your care.

- **Keep a list of all medicines you take.** Before taking your medicine, make sure it looks familiar. If it looks different from what you are accustomed to, ask questions.

- **Make sure you know the results of any test or procedure.** Ask your provider if you are unsure of the results.

- **Help remind your caregivers to wash their hands before they perform any "hands on" procedure.** Hand washing is important to prevent the spread of infection.

- **Make sure you understand what will happen if you have surgery.** You and your surgeon should agree clearly on what exactly needs to be done.

We invite you to share your ideas and suggestions about patient safety with us through our Patient Safety Suggestion Hotline: 232-1962.

HF-339 Rev. 1/03 ABQ

⊕LOVELACE

Source: Lovelace Health System, Albuquerque, New Mexico, 2003. Reprinted with permission.

Figure 3-3. Lovelace Health System Patient Safety Promise Card

---

Lovelace Health Systems is committed to providing safe patient care.

We invite you to ask questions at any time, or to share your suggestions about patient safety. Write your suggestions on this card or call our Hotline: 232-1962.

Patient Safety Suggestion: _____

_____
_____
_____
_____
_____
_____

Thank you for your suggestion. Please return this card to your nurse. Your nurse will forward them to our Patient Safety Program.

HF-368 2/03 ABQ

Source: Lovelace Health System, Albuquerque, New Mexico, 2003. Reprinted with permission.

- If potential problems are identified, the pharmacist recommends changes, and either the nurse or the pharmacist discusses the recommendations with the patient's physician.
- The nurse or the pharmacist educates the patient about changes in medications and the importance of continuing to update the medication card and bringing it to future clinic or hospital visits.

During Patient Safety Awareness week in May 2003, Lovelace Health System sponsored several patient-focused safety activities. For example, a special time was set aside for patients to bring in their medications and have a clinical pharmacist evaluate their medication regimen for interactions. Pharmacists also answered any questions patients might have had about their medications. At the same time, medication wallet cards were distributed to patients (figure 3-4). The pharmacists helped people fill in the card with the names of their prescription medicines, herbal and vitamin supplements, over-the-counter medicines, and allergy information. Patients were advised to keep the list up-to-date and to bring the card with them to each clinic or hospital visit. During Patient Safety Awareness week, Lovelace also sponsored two public presentations on medication safety and general safety in the home. Members of the organization's health plan received patient safety

Figure 3-4.   Lovelace Health System "Mark Your Meds" Card

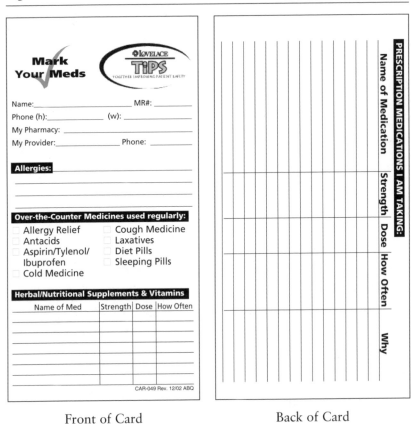

Front of Card   Back of Card

Source: Lovelace Health System, Albuquerque, New Mexico, 2002. Reprinted with permission.

information in the *Health & Fitness* and *Senior Health & Fitness* publications.

The University of Wisconsin (UW) Hospital and Clinics in Madison use other strategies to communicate the patient safety message to the public. One of the first projects, done in conjunction with the Madison Patient Safety Collaborative, was developing a consumer brochure called "Using Your Medications Safely: A Guide to Prescription Health."[43] This colorful eight-page pamphlet covers such topics as the following:

- Questions to ask your health care provider and pharmacist
- How to make the most of your visit to your health care provider
- How to make the most of your trip to the pharmacy
- Optimizing your medication use at home
- Maximizing medication safety when you are in the hospital
- Considerations for selecting a pharmacy

A medication wallet card is included in the brochure, as are instructions for using it effectively. The brochure is distributed to all patients at the time of hospital admission and used for education purposes by pharmacists and other caregivers. It is also available in all the clinic areas.

At the UW Hospital and Clinics, patients and families are very involved in medication reconciliation on admission and in learning about their medications on discharge. Each patient receives a medication interview from a pharmacist when admitted. If the patient is unable to communicate at the time of admission and family is not available, pharmacists routinely contact other sources (local pharmacies, physician offices, nursing homes, and so forth) to obtain information on medication use. At the time of discharge, a pharmacist provides medication teaching to the patient.

The UW Hospital and Clinics has also assembled an extensive library of patient education materials. Included in this library are fact sheets and brochures containing information on the role of patients and family members in making health care safer, such as the following:

- CT scans and safety
- Using restraints safely and why restraint use is limited as much as possible
- How to prevent falls

All patient education materials are reviewed and revised as needed at least every three years.

Posted in each patient room at the UW Hospital are tips on safety for patients and family members. In addition, caregivers encourage patients and their family to contact the patient relations department about any concerns, including matters related to patient safety. Feedback is used by the organization to make changes as appropriate. At the UW Children's Hospital, parent and adolescent advisory groups were formed several years ago to provide input into patient care issues including safety. Plans are under way to extend this advisory group concept to the adult population at the UW Hospital to ensure that patients and families are provided opportunities to proactively improve patient safety.

Several national groups have published strategies that providers can use to improve practitioner-patient partnerships. For example, in preparation for Patient Safety Awareness Week in 2003, the National Patient Safety Foundation prepared an extensive listing of activities for health care providers seeking to engage consumers in the patient safety movement.[44] These suggestions are found in figure 3-5. The ideas range from mass education campaigns to one-on-one knowledge-sharing opportunities. Education activities that are most effective are those that are personal and interactive between patients and caregivers. In these situations, the dialogue should go beyond knowledge building. Practitioners must emphasize behavior changes on the part of patients and families. Such exchanges will form the basis for a practitioner-patient partnership that promotes safety.

The "Quality Coach" column of the May 2003 issue of *Joint Commission: The Source*, published by the Joint Commission on Accreditation of Healthcare Organizations, outlined some strategies that health care team members can use during one-on-one interactions with patients to encourage their involvement in safety improvement. These recommendations are listed in figure 3-6.

Figure 3-5.   National Patient Safety Foundation Suggestions for Engaging Consumers in Patient Safety

Media and Marketing

- Tape a radio show on your local station about patient safety.
- Sponsor a resolution to declare the second week of March Patient Safety Awareness Week.
- Include a reminder about Patient Safety Awareness Week and safety tips with medical bills, paychecks.
- Distribute pins, pens, and other give-away items to "celebrate" your commitment to patient safety.
- Distribute press releases announcing your activities.
- Create public service announcements about communication, dialogue, and partnering between patients and health care providers. (To help get the message out, enlist major local radio and TV stations, along with university and local community print media, to provide in-kind support.)
- Write editorials, first-person stories, and op-ed pieces for local papers and newsletters.

Communicate and Partner with Patients and Families

- Offer a suggestion box for patients and families.
- Hold an open house, brown bag lunch, or roundtable discussion (with refreshments) for patients and families with a patient safety discussion.
- Hold a roundtable discussion with staff and patients and families to discuss safety concerns.
- Set up special phone lines for one week for consumers and staff to report safety concerns.
- Conduct surveys for the public to express their concerns about health care safety.
- Provide a journal or message board for patients to write down their stories and/or concerns while they are waiting for appointments.

Increase Patient Safety in Your Hospital or Organization

- Announce award programs and incentives.
- Hold a poster contest about patient safety.
- Provide a drop box for suggestions from staff to improve patient safety.
- Conduct a survey of staff about their safety concerns.
- Hold an information session about patient safety.
- Hold a roundtable discussion with staff to discuss safety concerns.
- Include patient safety in medical professional school curricula.
- Bring in a patient/family speaker to speak to staff about an experience with a medical error.
- Establish a Patient and Family Advisory Council in your hospital.

(Continued on next page)

Figure 3-5.   (Continued)

Educate Patients and Families

- Distribute literature in the lobby.
- Distribute medication safety pamphlets.
- Host a panel presentation and discussion.
- Invite speakers to come and speak about health care issues in hospital lobbies.
- Show educational films.
- Have a pharmacist available to answer questions in the lobby.
- Invite patients to bring their medications for review by a pharmacist.
- Empower patients by providing information on what they can do if they experience an error.

Provide Tools to Help Patients Ensure Their Own Care

- Distribute pillboxes with the days of the week, imprinted with a safety message and the name of the organizations.
- Distribute business cards or tent cards that read "Time to Clean Out Your Medicine Cabinet of Expired Medications" March 9–15, 2003.
- Distribute "My Personal Medical Diary" for patients to keep all of their records together, including medication, tests, and insurance. Encourage patients to know this information.
- Distribute wallet cards for patients to write down and carry with them all medications and phone numbers for providers and pharmacies.

Reach Out to the Community

- Introduce departments and services within your hospital to the patient and family population (such as ethics committees, social work, ombudsman programs, etc.).
- Use your volunteers, civic groups, and community groups to help pass out literature, write editorials, and post signs and posters throughout the community.
- Encourage educational and motivational speakers to go into businesses or to civic meetings (senior groups, PTAs, religious institutions) and speak about health care safety, or line them up for your own events!
- Hold an open house for civic groups and local residents to meet the staff, visit emergency rooms, and see your facility BEFORE they need it.
- Include a patient safety curriculum in high schools emphasizing "how to be an aware patient."

Reprinted with permission from the National Patient Safety Foundation®, Chicago [http://www.npsf.org/html/psaw.html]. Accessed July 2003.

Figure 3-6.   Strategies for Engaging Care Recipients in the Health Care Team

---

- Let individuals know that it's not only OK for them to ask questions but that you *expect* them to. Encourage care recipients to speak up if they don't understand what they've been told or what they should do.
- Use active communication, remembering the adage that a conversation is a two-way street. Ask questions that lead to discussion. For example, "Do you have any questions about your procedure?"
- Involve care recipients in all decisions about their care and treatment. Explain all options and the pros and cons of each option. Ask, "What are your thoughts about this treatment?"
- Enlist care recipients in the treatment process. Be honest and tell them that they can't leave it all up to their caregivers. You need their help to make treatment or care plans work.
- Encourage individuals to bring along a family member or friend who can act as their advocate.

© Joint Commission Resources, Joint Commission on Accreditation of Healthcare Organizations, Oakbrook Terrace, Ill., 2003. Reprinted with permission.

Source: Joint Commission Resources, "Engaging Care Recipients in the Health Care Team," *Joint Commission: The Source* 1, no. 5 (2003): 5.

Being Safe Together

> *Your Majesty, please . . . I don't like to complain,*
> *But down here below, we are feeling great pain.*
> *I know, up on top you are seeing great sights,*
> *But down at the bottom, we, too, should have rights.*
>
> —Theodore "Dr. Seuss" Geisel (Yertle)

There is overwhelming evidence that the safety of health care services can be improved. Although health care providers bear the major responsibility for reducing unintended medical errors, consumers can and should be encouraged to share responsibility for their own safety. There currently is insufficient evidence of the effectiveness of practitioner-patient partnerships in reducing adverse events, but common sense suggests that adding another safeguard—the patient—will not make matters worse. Some patients, fed up with what appears to be a national epidemic of medical misadventures, are demanding they be viewed as active error-prevention participants.

Consider the hindsight perspective of the nurse turned hospital patient for treatment of sepsis.

I was told that I would be discharged when the CT scan results had been called to the physician's office. There was a one-and-a-half-day administrative delay from the time of the physician's order for the CT scan until it was actually completed. When I returned from radiology, I got dressed in my street clothes and stood at the nurse's station waiting for my discharge instructions. One nurse looked at me and said, "Why are you dressed?" No one knew I was to go home that day.

An error that health care professionals have made over and over again is to think they know what the patient wants, feels, needs. However, we don't know and we can't know until we've been there. My experiences as a hospital patient made me realize that many health care professionals (including myself) lack the skills or desire needed to effectively partner with patients. Just a simple explanation of what to expect during my hospitalization, offered as soon as possible after my admission, would have reduced my anxieties. I wouldn't have been so quick to assume that things were going wrong, and I would have known when to speak up with valid concerns. Instead, I became the patient every health care professional dreads—constantly asking questions and seemingly never satisfied with the answers. By listening and learning from patients and their family members, we can realize significant safety improvements. The collaboration strategies and tools need not be expensive or difficult; they need only be used.

Health care providers and practitioners can create stronger partnerships with patients by building on past health care consumer education initiatives. This can be accomplished by validating that mistakes do occur in the delivery of health care services and then helping patients and families regain control (and self-esteem). Patients must be taught how to help themselves as they navigate the confusing and sometimes treacherous health care delivery system. In many instances, the patient is the only constant thread throughout the continuum of care. The patient's persistent and informed vigilance is a critical aspect of patient safety.

Most health care organizations have some components of patient safety already in place, and a few are aggressively involving patients and family members in error reduction activities. Health care organizations often have to overcome cultural barriers and outmoded attitudes before an outreach to patients and families can be successful. Once the patient safety mindset begins to take hold in the organization, it's time to create opportunities for consumer involvement in the patient safety movement. The most important consideration is that organizations start somewhere—whether it's staff training in active listening skills or organizationwide participation in Patient Safety Awareness Week activities. Partnering with consumers to improve the safety of health care services is not an event; it is a journey—a journey well worth taking.

References

1. A. Gawande, *Complications: A Surgeon's Notes on an Imperfect Science* (New York: Metropolitan Books, a division of Henry Holt and Company, 2002).
2. C. Perrow, *Normal Accidents: Living with High-Risk Technologies* (New York: Basic Books, 1984), 89–100.
3. American Hospital Association, Quality Advisory: "Improving Medication Safety by Partnering with Patients" (September 15, 2000).
4. Joint Commission on Accreditation of Healthcare Organizations "Speak Up" Campaign [http://www.jcaho.org/general+public/patient+safety/speak+up/speak+up.htm] (March 2002).
5. National Patient Safety Foundation, Chicago [http://www.npsf.org/html/patients.html#what]. Accessed May 2003.
6. National Council on Patient Information and Education [http://www.talkaboutrx.org/].
7. Agency for Healthcare Research and Quality, "AHRQ and National Council on Patient Information and Education Produce New Tool to Help Consumers Reduce Medication Errors" (press release) [http://www.ahcpr.gov/news/press/pr2003/safemedpr.htm] (April 30, 2003).
8. T. Bodenheimer, E. H. Wagner, and K. Grumbach, "Improving Primary Care for Patients with Chronic Illness," *Journal of the American Medical Association* 288, no. 14 (2002): 1775–79.

9. L. T. Kohn, J. M. Corrigan, and M. S. Donaldson, eds., *To Err Is Human: Building a Safer Health System*, Institute of Medicine Committee on Quality of Health Care in America (Washington, D.C.: National Academy Press, 1999), 150.

10. American College of Physicians, "The Role of the Patient in Patient Safety" [http://www.acponline.org/ptsafety/patient.htm]. Accessed June 2003.

11. The Minnesota Alliance for Patient Safety, "Patient Safety: Your Role" [http://www.mhhp.com/patientsafety/patientsafety.pdf] (2002).

12. National Patient Safety Foundation, "National Agenda for Action: Patients and Families in Patient Safety: *Nothing About Me, Without Me*" (2003) [http://www.npsf.org/download/AgendaFamilies.pdf]. Accessed June 2003.

13. C. Edwards, "A Proposal That Patients Be Considered Honorary Members of the Healthcare Team," *Journal of Clinical Nursing* 11, no. 3 (May 2002): 340–48.

14. N. K. G Mendis, ed., *The Questions of King Milinda: Abr't of Milindapanha* (Seattle, Wash.: Pariyatti Press, 1993).

15. M. A. LaCombe, "On Bedside Teaching," *Annals of Internal Medicine* 126 (1997): 217–20.

16. M. E. Knowles, *The Modern Practice of Adult Education* (Englewood Cliffs, N.J.: Cambridge/Prentice Hall, 1980), 43–44.

17. B. Nair, J. Coughlan, and M. Hensley, "Student and Patient Perspectives on Bedside Teaching," *Medical Education* 31 (1997): 341–46.

18. P. N. Uhlig and others, "Reconfiguring Clinical Teamwork for Safety and Effectiveness," *Focus on Patient Safety* 5 (2002): 1–2.

19. The Bayer Institute for Health Care Communication [http://www.bayerinstitute.com].

20. American Academy of Orthopaedic Surgeons, *1999 Public Image Investigation. Second Report* (Rosemont, Ill.: American Academy of Orthopaedic Surgeons, May 1999).

21. American Academy of Orthopaedic Surgeons, Communication Skills Mentoring Program [http://www3.aaos.org/courses/csmp/index.htm]. Accessed May 2003.

22. J. R. Tongue, "Patient Encounter Tips," AAOS Communication Skills Mentoring Program [http://www3.aaos.org/courses/csmp/Initialed Encounter.htm]. Accessed May 2003.

23. Personal correspondence between Patrice Spath and Dr. John Tongue, May 26, 2003.

24. A. Mehrabian, *Silent Messages* (Belmont, Calif.: Wadsworth, 1971).

25. M. Pickering, "Communication," *Explorations: A Journal of Research of the University of Maine* 3, no. 1 (1986): 16–19.

26. J. Conway, "Tools for Patient Safety," presentation at the 2001 User Liaison Program, "Beyond State Reporting: Medical Errors and

Patient Safety Issues," sponsored by the Agency for Healthcare Research and Quality, Nashville, Tenn.

27. G. Sprenger, "Deal to Tell It All," presentation at the 3rd Annenberg Conference on Patient Safety, St. Paul, Minn., 2001.

28. J. Morath, "Changing the Culture of Patient Safety," presentation at the BJC HealthCare Patient Safety Forum, St. Louis, Mo., 2003.

29. K. Davis and others, *Room for Improvement: Patient Reports on the Quality of Their Health Care* (New York: The Commonwealth Fund, April 2002).

30. Virginians Improving Patient Care and Safety, "Be Involved in Your Health Care," Richmond, Va. [http://www.vipcs.org]. Accessed June 2003.

31. Agency for Healthcare Research and Quality [http://www.ahrq.gov/consumer/].

32. Institute for Safe Medication Practices [www.ismp.org].

33. National Patient Safety Foundation, "You Can Improve Patient Safety" [http://www.npsf.org/html/patients.html]. Accessed June 2003.

34. National Patient Safety Foundation, "National Patient Safety Awareness Week" [http://www.npsf.org/html/psaw.html]. Accessed June 2003.

35. Joint Commission on Accreditation of Healthcare Organizations, "Speak Up: Help Prevent Errors in Your Care" [http://www.jcaho.org/general+public/patient+safety/speak+up/index.htm]. Accessed June 2003.

36. PULSE America [http://www.pulseamerica.org].

37. Parents of Infants and Children with Kernicterus [http://www.pick online.org/index.html].

38. M. J. Field and K. N. Lohr, eds., *Guidelines for Clinical Practice: From Development to Use*, Committee on Clinical Practice Guidelines, Institute of Medicine (Washington, D.C.: National Academy Press, 1992), 83–88.

39. Ibid., 88.

40. L. T. Pizzi, N. I. Goldfarb, and D. B. Nash, "Other Practices Related to Patient Participation," in *Making Health Care Safer: A Critical Analysis of Patient Safety Practices* (Rockville, Md.: Agency for Healthcare Research and Quality, U.S. Department of Health and Human Services, July 20, 2001) (AHRQ Publication 01-E058).

41. Field and Lohr, *Guidelines for Clinical Practice*, 88.

42. J. Williamson, "Medical Quality Management Systems in Perspective," in *Health Care Quality Management for the 21st Century*, ed. J. Couch (Tampa, Fla.: American College of Physician Executives, 1991).

43. This brochure is available on the Web site of the Madison Patient Safety Collaborative [http://www.madisonpatientsafety.org].

44. National Patient Safety Foundation, "National Patient Safety Awareness Week" [http://www.npsf.org/html/psaw.html]. Accessed June 2003.

4

Engaging Patients in Safety: Barriers and Solutions

Michelle H. Pelling, M.B.A., R.N.

Health care consumers have a legitimate interest in their own safety. For this reason, many patients are becoming acculturated to the need for actively participating in their own care. At most stages of health care, there is the potential for patients to contribute to their own care through the provision of pertinent health information, participation in the plan of care and treatment decisions, and self-management of their condition. Researchers have documented that patient participation in the health care experience can lead to better outcomes, fewer disease-related limitations, more efficient use of resources, and improved patient satisfaction.[1] Moreover, active involvement by patients in their own care is vital because patient knowledge, self-observation, and feedback to the providers are routinely needed for sound medical decision making. The effect of active patient and family involvement on reducing medical errors is still under investigation; however, anecdotal results are promising.[2]

Provision of safe health care services is an objective for every health care provider. It is in everyone's best interests to prevent untoward side effects, treatment-related injuries, communication failures, and technical mishaps. Active involvement of patients in the health care experience provides another safety check in health care processes. By paying attention to the care being provided to them, patients can alert caregivers to potential errors so that corrective actions can be initiated before any harm occurs. For purposes of patient safety improvement, it is incumbent on all providers to embrace patients and family members as active participants on the health care team.

85

How Patients Can Help

Patients can help health care professionals do their jobs safely and protect themselves from harmful mistakes by taking the following actions:

- Talking with caregivers—telling about their history, problems they have had in the past, medications they have been taking, what is confusing to them, and what concerns they may have

- Reminding caregivers to confirm their identity before administering any medication or treatment and by speaking up if it appears the caregiver has them confused with someone else

- Confirming that caregivers know what the doctor has ordered for them and that the caregivers have all the information needed in order to provide safe care

- Telling caregivers about their allergies to any medications or food and reminding everyone to communicate information about their allergies to food and medications to other members of the health care team

- Informing caregivers if they have been taking any medicinal herbal products or over-the-counter medications, which can help prevent unnecessary drug-to-drug or drug-to-food interactions and adverse drug reactions

- Giving caregivers any medications they have brought to the hospital from home so that potential interactions with other medications or other injuries can be prevented

- Asking caregivers to explain the medications that are being offered to verify if it is the right medication for them; if not, questioning the caregiver's decision to administer the medication

- Asking questions about their care plan so that they fully understand what they need to do and how they should do it, including how to change dressings and the frequency and dosage of their medications

- Telling their surgeon or anesthesia professional about all of their health conditions, allergic reactions, and the medications they take
- Asking hospital staff members if they have reviewed the history and physical report that was provided by their primary doctor or surgeon
- Asking questions about the risks involved with anesthesia and/or medications they will receive during a surgery or a procedure
- Reminding caregivers to mark the site of the procedure so there is no confusion in the operating room or procedure area and verifying that everyone knows where the procedure will be performed
- Asking caregivers to explain why a test or treatment may be needed and how it might help them in order to identify an incorrect order for a test or a test that is meant for another patient
- Asking about test results, what they mean, and how they will be addressed
- Asking about the equipment used in their care to understand what different sounds or noises mean so they can notify caregivers if it appears there may be a potential problem[3]

Active patient involvement is the right thing to do, but this goal can be difficult to achieve. As the primary beneficiaries of health care services (and the recipients of any medical errors), patients, it would seem, have the most to gain from improvements in safety. Yet practitioners may find it challenging to engage patients and family members in error prevention activities; some people appear satisfied to remain uninvolved and uninformed. There are also barriers that originate from health care professionals themselves. Patriarchal attitudes, ineffective communication skills, and perceived lack of time are just some of the impediments to helping patients become active participants in their own care. The common barriers on both sides of the patient-practitioner partnership are discussed in this chapter along with strategies for reducing these obstacles.

The Empowered Patient

Improving the safety of health care services may depend in part on the patient's active involvement; some people, however, may not wish to be involved. Patients may be unaccustomed to active participation in health services delivery and consequently don't expect their caregivers to encourage them to do otherwise. Other patients are more demanding and critical of the care they receive. These people are offended when they are not treated as equal members of the health care team. Most patients are somewhere between these two extremes. The challenge for health care professionals is to understand how best to recognize and respond to the desires of the individual patient.

Factors Affecting the Degree of Patient Cooperation

Put yourself in the place of a newly hospitalized patient. You feel miserable and frightened. The nurse asks your family to wash their hands each time they visit and also mentions that you should remind nurses to do the same thing in case they forget. Now, in addition to feeling miserable and frightened, you're confused. You may find yourself wondering, "Shouldn't my nurses always remember to wash their hands before touching me? I wonder what else they might forget to do?"

Inviting patients to be involved in safety reveals to them the risk of errors. Some patients will choose to shoulder responsibility for safer health care delivery, whereas others will be content to sit back and rely on health care professionals to do it right every time. A number of factors contribute to patients' willingness to share safety improvement responsibilities.

Preoccupation with Other Issues

Patients may be wrestling with internal or external constraints that inhibit effective communication with practitioners. Patients may be worrying about family or employment issues or coping with a new diagnosis. They may be anxious about financial difficulties or may have unresolved personal matters. A patient that doesn't respond positively to suggestions for more active participation in the health care experience may very well be interested in participating but needs time to deal with personal issues first.

Fear

Some patients may not voice concerns about safety for fear of offending health care providers. In the past, caregivers may have rebuked the patient when he or she spoke up about unsafe situations or questioned health care practices. Health care professionals often tell patients not to worry and to put more trust in their providers. This can create a situation in which patients think their concerns won't be listened to or it won't do any good to express them. Some patients are fearful that raising questions might actually cause an error to occur or think their question is not legitimate. Especially in situations where patients feel vulnerable, they don't want to be viewed by caregivers as being too demanding.

Denial

Although there has been considerable media attention on medical errors, patients often believe that an error won't happen to them. They have an almost blind faith in the ability of health care professionals to not make mistakes. Patients frequently don't appreciate that mistakes are often caused by breakdowns in the process of care, something that competent professionals can't always control. And even competent practitioners are fallible.

Indifference

Some patients resent being asked to participate in protecting themselves from mistakes that might be made during the delivery of health services. It's not uncommon to hear a patient say, "It is their job to take care of me; that's what they are getting paid for!" The traditional paternalistic attitude of health care professionals has contributed in no small way to this indifference.[4] All too often patients were—and are—expected to be passive and dependent rather than active coproducers of health care services.

Age and Condition

Some studies of patient participation in health care decision making suggest that older, sicker patients are more likely than others to be passive.[5] Unfortunately, these are the patients who stand to benefit the most from error prevention strategies because their care is usually complex and likely to involve multiple caregivers and sites of care. Older patients are typically not accustomed to being active health care participants and become anxious when practitioners encourage them to speak up. Younger patients tend to be more assertive; however, this attitude can change to passivity if the patient is faced with a life-threatening disease.

Education and Literacy

It is estimated that up to 90 million patients in the United States have some type of health illiteracy that negatively impacts their understanding of health care information. A recent study, for example, indicates that up to 40 percent of the people surveyed (the respondents) were unable to fully understand the information and warnings contained on a common prescription bottle.[6] Even people who can sign their names may lack the skills needed to assimilate verbal or written instructions communicated by caregivers. Patients with low literacy often feel embarrassed and therefore may not ask questions or reveal that they don't understand.

Language

English is not the primary language for many patients. Interpreters may be present for the diagnostic or treatment interactions with clinicians, but these are not always the ideal times for communicating information about safety. Written materials used to educate patients about their role in maintaining a safe environment can be confusing or misleading if translated literally into other languages.

Culture

Patients come from a wide variety of ethnic groups with diverse religious, social, and cultural beliefs. In some societies, it would be considered bad manners for the physician or nurse to ask the patient or family members to assist in preventing mistakes, so merely asking a patient to express safety concerns may not yield a satisfactory response. In many cultures, patients and family members accept the physician's decision or the nurse's direction without question. Patients may not be accustomed to making choices about their own health needs and would never think to point out a mistake that has been made. Stressful situations, such as a serious illness, can lead to even greater patient-practitioner communication difficulties.

Strengthening Patient Involvement

Questions that must be asked: Do consumers *want* to be involved in the patient safety movement? To what extent is such an agenda paternalistic (i.e., guardians looking after the best interests of the consumers) and to what extent is it truly consumer driven? Past studies of patients' interest in shared health care decision making may provide a clue. There is compelling evidence to suggest that patient involvement in health care decisions has a positive effect on patient satisfaction, compliance with treatment recommendations, and outcomes.[7] For this reason, models of patient care that emphasize the patient's active involvement are being promoted. Researchers have discovered that some patients want to play no role in the decision process, and yet others want to take full control in the therapy selection.[8] Most studies suggest that only a minority of patients wish to assume the role of primary decision maker.

It is quite likely the same variation will be found when consumers are asked about being involved in the prevention of medical errors. Some people will express the belief that health care providers should have sufficient knowledge and skills to prevent mistakes, and health care processes should be designed more safely. These people expect providers to function as the sole guardians of safety. Other consumers will accept information about their role in preventing medical errors but may not act on the information unless providers are supportive. For these people, health care professionals must function in the role of friend or teacher to encourage their involvement. For action to occur, both the consumer and provider must believe that the patient's active participation can have a positive impact on safety.

A third group of consumers deliberately seek out information on medical error prevention. These consumers may have personally experienced a medical mishap and wish to deter future problems, or they may be fearful of a mistake because of media reports or discussions with friends or relatives.[9] Medical-error prevention information may be obtained directly from providers or other sources (e.g., consumer groups, medical professional associations, Internet health sites, support groups). Even though these patients may have a limited understanding of clinical care and associated processes, they may try to oversee all aspects of health care safety. Some providers view this group of consumers as "meddlers," which unfortunately can widen the patient-practitioner communication gap. Caregivers have a responsibility to assist proactive consumers in accessing, understanding, and applying the information they need to be more effective partners with the health care team.

One would presume that all consumers would embrace the opportunity to prevent health services errors that might cause personal harm. However, a recent study of patient participation in surgery-site marking confirmed that many people would choose a passive role. Researchers discovered that a surprisingly high number (35 percent) did not comply with the orthopedist's request to mark "NO" on the extremity that was not to be operated on, even when patients were told that such a mark was intended to prevent wrong-site surgery. The researchers concluded that patients undergoing surgery must be encouraged to take a more active role in their health care in order to optimize outcomes and minimize risks.[10]

Patients cannot participate in safety improvement activities unless they have the right types of information, given in ways optimal for their own level of understanding. There is a compelling need for education and other interventions to communicate with consumers about how to improve the safety of their health care experience. True patient participation in safety requires that health care professionals have an awareness of patient expectations and perceived needs and the extent to which these needs are being adequately addressed.

Practice Implications

What does such awareness mean to health care professionals? For one thing, it doesn't mean that practitioners should give up on their attempts to involve patients and their families in the patient safety movement. That would be irresponsible. Understanding the barriers to effective patient-practitioner partnerships is the first step toward designing better ways of encouraging and educating patients, especially those prone to passivity, to become active members of the health care team. The following strategies have proved successful.

Use Your Position

The status of health care professionals in the eyes of patients can be a benefit. Most patients, respectful of their physicians, nurses, and other caregivers, will respond well to an invitation to help out. By saying something like "I will do my job better if you read this material or follow these suggestions," the clinician is inviting the patient to help make his or her job easier. This approach encourages patients (and family members) to be involved with the practitioner in delivering safe care.

During the delivery of care, practitioners should serve as models for safe behaviors and point out what is being done for safety purposes. When the doctor states, "I'm checking your allergies before I prescribe this medication," the patient can see that even competent practitioners need reminders on occasion to prevent slipups. Patients will also realize the importance of sharing information about their allergies; otherwise, caregivers won't be able to do their job as effectively.

Facilitating patient participation in error reduction activities requires a time commitment from caregivers. The most anxiety-producing aspect of the patient-practitioner relationship is lack of time. If the caregiver doesn't allow sufficient time to discuss various strategies for reducing mistakes, the patient may be left with the nagging fear that safety is not a high priority for the provider. The basic problem is the time that effective communication requires. The rapid pace of health care, especially in acute care settings, can impede communication. Concern for other patients and the tasks that need to be completed can cause health care professionals to become distracted and listen with only partial attention. Fatigue, stress, and anxiety that often stem from poor communication with other care providers, cumbersome information systems, and confusing protocols and procedures create barriers to spending time listening to patients and exploring their questions and concerns.[11] All of these pressures make health care professionals poor communication role models for patients.

How practitioners interact with patients can have a dramatic effect on whether patients are comfortable speaking up. Patients may be reluctant to raise issues or talk about concerns if they sense that the caregiver is uncomfortable or doesn't have time to engage in the discussion. This happens when health care professionals use "blocking behaviors" that discourage continued discussion.[12] Examples of blocking behaviors are listed in figure 4-1.

Patients learn a great deal about how to communicate with health care professionals by watching how practitioners interact with them. When clinicians model positive communication traits, those same traits can be cultivated in patients. Patients won't respond to an invitation to become an active health care participant simply because the practitioner tells them to. Patients want and deserve explanations about safety. When caregivers don't take sufficient time to explain, patients may begin to doubt the providers' commitment to keeping them safe.

Relinquish Paternalism

In ancient times, medicine was based on magic and religion. The divine Greco-Roman god of medicine, Aesculopius, was worshipped in hundreds of temples throughout Greece. The sick gathered at these temples for a healing ritual known as "incubation" or "temple sleep." While in a dream state, the sick were visited by Aesculopius or one of his priests who gave advice. According to ancient writings, many patients, on awakening, were cured of their ailments.

The science of medicine has changed considerably since Roman times, although for centuries patients continued to be denied credibility or authority over their treatment, presumably because they were seen as "too sick" to be listened to. Attempts to guide patient decisions often tended toward paternalism rather than genuine empowerment. It wasn't until the last half of the 20th century

Figure 4-1.   Blocking Behaviors That Inhibit Practitioner-Patient Communication

- Defend an action we have taken and block patients from continuing to express their concern.
- Interrupt and finish sentences of patients, cutting them off before they are able to express their concern in their own words.
- Talk more than patients—making it difficult for them to squeeze their perspective into the conversation.
- Deliberately change the subject because we are uncomfortable. This shuts down everyone, except the most persistent patient, from being able to express concerns.
- Fail to clarify patients' concerns and run the risk of misunderstanding what they have said and taking an inappropriate course of action.
- Offer premature or inappropriate reasons or answers. We may be acting on too little information and misadvise patients. In these situations, patients may feel their concerns are being invalidated.
- Cite policy as the reason for an action. This communicates to the patient that only hospital policy matters, not his or her needs or feelings.
- Overtly avoid an issue. This communicates a lack of interest in the patient's concern and often shuts down dialogue with the patient on other issues. This is a definite disincentive for the patient to speak up again.
- Minimize the patient's concern. Patients may lose face or feel they have overreacted or were just plain silly for speaking up at all.
- Disregard the patient's concern with condescending comments such as "We have got it handled." This conveys disrespect for the patient's feelings and concerns.
- Make promises to do things we don't or can't follow through on. This jeopardizes the patient's confidence and trust in everyone on the health care team.
- Put down the organization. This causes a loss of the patient's trust in our ability to care for him or her safely. It compromises any respect we have been able to build with the patient.

that consumers in some countries, including the United States, started to demand a more active and personal role in the health care experience.[13]

Broad societal changes have shifted the demands, expectations, and attitudes of health care consumers. Old-style paternalism, for all its achievements, is now a barrier to patient safety. Patients want caregivers who will be counselors and interpreters, not just guardians of knowledge.[14] Once health care professionals relinquish paternalistic attitudes, they are forced to develop and enhance their repertoire of communication skills: listening to patients, answering questions, helping patients make decisions, directing patients to appropriate resource materials, and being fellow learners.

Health care professionals often don't appreciate how patients can help prevent errors. The author informally polled physicians, nurses, and other health care professionals at five different hospitals to ascertain their views on patient involvement in the safety movement. She discovered that many practitioners thought patients and their families don't have the knowledge or ability to contribute to their own safety because laypersons are unable to fully comprehend the technical aspects of health care. Some hospital nurses expressed concerns that constant questions or reminders voiced by patients will interfere with nurses' performing their work. Some nurses believed that asking patients to bring up safety concerns was more of a "customer service" than an intervention that would actually help reduce errors.

By now you may have heard the cliché describing the changing role of the health care practitioner from "a sage on the stage to a guide on the side." To effectively partner with consumers in the patient safety movement, health care professionals must become consultants, advisers, and confidantes. Fortunately, evidence in recent years is showing that many health service providers are increasingly recognizing the importance of patient participation, which involves listening to, and acting on, advice from patients. From the perspective of safety, health care consumers are in a unique position to identify problems and suggest solutions based on experiential knowledge.

Communicate from the Patient's Perspective

Effective communication is necessary if patients and their families are to become involved in preventing medical mishaps. Communication breakdowns can be caused by language differences and verbal misunderstandings as well as by cultural differences. Language differences may be easy to compensate for, but it is equally important—and perhaps more difficult—to overcome cultural barriers. A little knowledge, a lot of alertness, and the willingness to work within another person's cultural norms can go far toward creating better patient-practitioner partnerships.

All consumer materials related to patient safety should be available in the person's native language. This may seem an obvious suggestion for the non-English-speaking patient, but often health care professionals fail to recognize that people who can speak English may not be able to read English or may prefer reading in their own language. If English is a patient's second language, it is important to determine the patient's English proficiency and offer bilingual patient safety materials or interpreters. Many of the patient safety consumer education materials developed by the Agency for Healthcare Research and Quality are available in English and Spanish.[15] Organizations such as Harborview Medical Center in Seattle, Washington, have developed multilingual patient education materials.[16]

The value of practitioner sensitivity to cultural barriers cannot be underestimated. An important factor as it relates to patient safety is that 75 percent of cultures around the world are group oriented. One of the many manifestations of this cultural value is the extreme importance of the extended family. Family members want to be involved in the patient's care and, if educated about safety along with the patient, can greatly increase the likelihood that the information will be retained and practiced. There are numerous other issues to consider when caring for patients from other ethnic groups; however, the topic is well beyond the scope of this chapter. A number of resources to assist health care professionals in understanding how to interact with patients from various cultures are listed in figure 4-2.

Figure 4-2.   Cultural Diversity Resources for Health Care
Professionals

*Volunteers in Health Care Guide to Cross Cultural Communications
for Health Care Organizations.* Available free online at:
www.volunteersinhealthcare.org, or by calling 877-844-8442.

Ethnomedicine Information Web site sponsored by Harborview Medical
Center, Seattle, Wash.: http://www.ethnomed.org.

Multi-Lingual Health Education Net. This Web site sponsored by a
group of British Columbia health agencies contains high-quality
translated information for healthcare providers and their clients:
http://www.multilingual-health-education.net.

Center for Cross-Cultural Health sponsored by the University of
Minnesota: http://www.crosshealth.com.

Rachael E. Spector. *Cultural Diversity in Health and Illness,* 5th ed.
(Upper Saddle River, N.J.: Prentice Hall, 2000).

Geri-Ann Galanti. *Caring for Patients from Different Cultures: Case
Studies from American Hospitals,* 2nd ed. (Philadelphia: University of
Pennsylvania Press, 1997).

The Western Journal of Medicine 157, no. 3 (September 1992). Special
issue on Cross-Cultural Medicine.

David V. Espino, ed. *Clinics in Geriatric Medicine: Ethnogeriatrics*
(Philadelphia: W. B. Saunders Co., 1995).

"Cultural Competence and Care Recipient Safety," *Joint Commission
Perspectives on Patient Safety* 22, no. 2 (February 2002).

Literacy also affects patient-practitioner communication.
Patients with low literacy can misunderstand verbal or written
communications. Recognizing this as problematic, the U.S. Department of Health and Human Services mandated in its "Healthy People 2010" report that all health care communications designed for
patients be scrutinized for an appropriate reading comprehension
level. In this case, *appropriate* is defined as the reading comprehension level congruent with the reading level of the majority of
patients. Too often, printed materials baffle patients because authors
don't take into account the users' literacy level, reading skills,
thinking style, or short-term memory.

All written patient safety education materials should be tested for readability. One way is to use readability software to make sure the target population can read the booklets. But writing at a lower-grade level may not be more understandable if some of the other issues, such as type size and line length, aren't addressed. An even better idea is to ask patients and family members to help evaluate and rewrite the materials.

Keep Patients Informed

Patients are frequently told to speak up when they have a concern. Yet how many patients know the difference between what should be happening and what is *actually* happening? For patients to serve as effective system safeguards, it is vital for them to know more about the health care process. For example, clinic patients should be told when to expect to hear back from their physician (or their designee) about diagnostic test results.

The patient should be told to initiate contact with the physician if no communication has been received within a specified period. Patients may believe that "no news is good news" when, in fact, test results may have never been delivered to the physician. The missing results fell through the cracks in the system. The patient-initiated contact with the physician might possibly be the last line of defense in making sure test results get to the right place.

Some hospitals have created informational brochures or patient education tools that explain what will happen during hospitalization. An example of a patient version of a clinical path is shown in figure 4-3. The clinical path describes in layperson terms what is most likely to happen during the hospital stay for a laparoscopic cholecystectomy. A nurse from the hospital's day surgery unit uses this document as a teaching tool during preadmission patient education. Armed with a better understanding of what is likely to happen, patients can now become active participants. It is easier for patients or family members to speak up when something doesn't seem quite right if they know what to expect. Providing process transparency, where it makes sense, allows patients to be more involved in error prevention.

Figure 4-3. Patient Version of a Clinical Path for Laparoscopic Cholecystectomy

Before Admission	Before Surgery	After Surgery	At Discharge
Your doctor will do a medical history and physical and have you sign a form giving him/her permission to do surgery.	An anesthesiologist will talk with you and discuss the type of anesthesia to be used for your surgery.		Your physician or the surgical resident assisting him/her will see you before you are discharged.
A nurse from the hospital's day-surgery unit will call you the day before surgery. The nurse will tell you: • What time to arrive at the hospital • Not to eat or drink anything the night before surgery • What medications to take the night before, or morning of, surgery • To have someone available to take you home	Your blood pressure, pulse, respirations, and temperature will be taken when you arrive. An intravenous line will be started in your vein and you will receive an antibiotic. You will be asked to empty your bladder 5 to 10 minutes before going to surgery.	The nurse will monitor your blood pressure, pulse, breathing, and temperature frequently. If you have any discomfort, ask your nurse for some medication. You should empty your bladder 4 to 6 hours after your surgery. If you can't empty your bladder or feel uncomfortable, tell your nurse. Your intravenous line will be removed when you are drinking enough fluids.	

			You will receive instructions on: • Activity at home • Diet • Medications • Follow-up appointment • Symptoms to report to your doctor • Wound care
Your doctor and day-surgery nurse at the hospital will explain the procedure to be done and your care after the surgery. You may need some tests done before your surgery.	You will need to arrive at the hospital 1½ hours before your scheduled surgery. A nurse will teach you about leg exercises and how to cough and take deep breaths after surgery.	You will be reminded to do your breathing exercises. You can begin to drink clear liquids and eat when you feel you are ready.	You will be ready for discharge as soon as you have emptied your bladder, are able to tolerate oral intake, and can walk with assistance.
Let the nurse know if there is no one at home to help you after surgery.	If you have any questions, the nurse and doctor or resident will answer them for you. You will be asked if you have a ride home when you are discharged.	You will begin to receive discharge instructions.	

Source: Patrice Spath, *Mastering Path-Based Patient Care* (Forest Grove, Ore.: Brown-Spath & Associates, 1995). Reprinted with permission.

Widespread support is given to the idea that the partnership between practitioners and patients should be improved and strengthened. Furnishing better and timely information to patients is an essential element of health service safety. A revolutionary way of keeping patients informed about the health care experience has begun in the United Kingdom. This initiative involves providing patients with copies of clinician-to-clinician letters and is intended as a way to increase patients' involvement in their care and treatment and keep them up-to-date on all matters related to their health.

A common complaint by patients is that doctors and nurses talk about them as if they weren't there. So why should clinicians correspond with one another about patients without including the patients in the information loop? Supporters of the United Kingdom initiative suggest that copying letters to patients involves them more personally in their care.[17] Commenting in support of the project, Harry Cayton, director of Patient Experience and Public Involvement, United Kingdom Department of Health, noted that the new relationship between health professionals and service users requires openness, mutual respect, sharing of expertise, and joint decision making. Copying physicians' letters to patients is one small step on the way to rebalancing the patient-practitioner relationship—but a symbolic and important one.[18] The response of health care consumers in the United Kingdom has been very positive. A patient from one of the pilot sites for copying letters to patients said: "It lets you know what the hospital knows. There should be no secrets, no constraints—generally, I thought it was brilliant. In the past you didn't get to know anything. You walked into the hospital grounds not knowing anything."[19]

There are, of course, practical matters to be considered in copying letters to patients: patient consent, the ability of practitioners to be technically precise while reasonably comprehensible, security, and confidentiality. These issues are not insurmountable, but it would be unfortunate if health care professionals were unwilling to tackle the issues merely because copying letters to patients might require a change in usual health service work practices.[20]

Education and knowledge are empowering forces for patients wishing to take an active role in the health care experience, and providers must support this role. Carl Carpenter, Ph.D., a member of the board at The Regional Medical Center in Orangeburg, South Carolina, feels strongly that hospitals must become more involved in creating partnerships with patients. "Physicians, nurses, and other health care providers have to become better 'facilitators of learning' for patients, and we've got to support that transition. Trustees should be asking: 'What can our hospital do to help strengthen patient-caregiver collaboration?'"[21]

Be Open and Honest

Health care professionals can work in partnership with patients in a number of ways. By offering explanations about procedures that will be performed, medications that will be administered, or other activities to be conducted, practitioners are giving patients an opportunity to act as a safeguard in the process. Patient-practitioner dialogue cannot be just one-sided. There should be a back-and-forth exchange of information. And this means that it is hoped patients will communicate their safety concerns to practitioners. To maintain open dialogue with patients, caregivers must be adequately prepared to respond when one of those patients says, "I think you may have made a mistake." Such statements can cause clinicians to become defensive and seek ways of disengaging or discrediting the discussion. Drs. Chassin and Becker described this phenomenon in an article about the case of a patient who was mistakenly taken for another patient's invasive electrophysiology procedure. Despite the patient's repeated objections, the practitioners discounted what the patient was saying. The physicians and nurses believed the patient lacked information about the planned procedure.[22]

Health care activities are often very confusing to patients, so it's reasonable that patients or family members may perceive a situation inaccurately. In addition, how caregivers respond to inquiries influences patients' willingness to voice other concerns. If a mistake has not been made, caregivers should explain the situation because it's important to acknowledge the validity of patients' concerns and apologize for any confusion or lack of communication that may have occurred. Caregivers should thank patients and families for paying attention and congratulate them for asking questions. Encourage patients to speak up again by explaining that mistakes sometimes do occur and it is helpful for them to be vigilant.

If a patient's inquiry results in the realization that a mistake has been made, caregivers must take responsibility, apologize, and act to mitigate or correct the error or concern. Do not be defensive when this situation occurs. The patient-practitioner dialogue should go something like this: "Thank you for telling me. I'm sorry this happened, and I understand why you are upset. This is what I am going to do about it. I will get back to you in a little while and make sure everything has been resolved."

Reducing errors is a major challenge for health care organizations. The practitioner's response to patients' questions, concerns, and feedback will directly influence how willing patients are to assist in preventing or intercepting errors.

Working Together for Safety

Studies suggest that consumer faith and confidence in the medical profession has been eroding in the United States as well as in many other Western nations. Growing consumer skepticism about the quality and safety of patient care will lead toward less deferential, more informed, and more demanding patients. If health care professionals want to enlist the help of patients in preventing medical mistakes, new patient-practitioner relationships must be formed.

It should be no surprise that *Marcus Welby, M.D.*, was one of the most popular doctor shows in American television history. During the 1970 television year, it ranked number one among all TV series.[23] The scripts, authored by writer-physician Michael Halberstam, portrayed an idealized doctor-patient relationship characterized by Welby's incredibly solicitous and loyal bedside manner. Welby's demeanor undoubtedly influenced the public's image of the ideal practitioner. Some members of the medical profession even claimed that Welby was among the factors contributing to the rise of malpractice actions against physicians in the 1970s.[24]

To effectively engage health care consumers in safety improvement, it is not necessary for health care professionals to be just like Dr. Welby. However, patients and their families do expect to be reassured, supported, and provided with adequate explanations. Practitioners must reach out to the patient and the patient's family to involve them in issues of safety to the extent that they are capable or merely wish to be involved.

Greater understanding about the risks inherent in the health care system is fundamentally useful for patients. If patient education is to make a difference in the safety of health services, however, practitioners must understand and overcome barriers that can undermine the value of patient involvement. No one has more interest in health care safety than patients. Health care professionals must accept patients as partners, trust their expertise, and allow them to help transform health care into a safer system.

References

1. S. Greenfield, S. Kaplan, and J. E. Ware, "Expanding Patient Involvement: Effects on Patient Outcomes," *Annals of Internal Medicine* 102 (1985): 520–28; D. M. Vickery and others, "The Effect of Self-Care Interventions on the Use of Medical Services within a Medicare Population," *Medical Care* 26 (1988): 580–88; D. Brody and others, "Patient Perception of Involvement in Medical Care: Relationship to Illness Attitudes and Outcomes," *Journal of General Internal Medicine* 4, no. 6 (1989): 506–11; P. D. Mullen, "Compliance Becomes Concordance," *British Medical Journal* 314 (1997): 691.

2. S. A. Weigman and M. R. Cohen, "The Patient's Role in Preventing Medication Errors," in *Medication Errors,* ed. M. Cohen (Washington, D.C.: American Pharmaceutical Association, 2002); E. J. Sobo and others, "Rapid Interview Protocol Supporting Patient-Centered Quality Improvement: Hearing the Parent's Voice in a Pediatric Care Unit," *Joint Commission Journal of Quality Improvement* 28 (2002): 498–509.

3. M. H. Pelling, *Staying Safe: Your Role in the Healthcare Environment* (video) (Carrollton, Tx.: PRIMEDIA Healthcare, a division of PRIMEDIA Workplace Learning, 2001).

4. C. Laine and F. Davidoff, "Patient-Centered Medicine: A Professional Evolution," *Journal of the American Medical Association* 275 (1996): 152–56.

5. A. M. Stiggelbout and M. Gwendoline, "A Role of the Sick Patient: Patient Preferences Regarding Information and Participation in Clinical Decision-Making," *Canadian Medical Association Journal* 157, no. 4 (1997): 383–89.

6. J. Moisan and others, "Non-compliance with Drug Treatment and Reading Difficulties with Regard to Prescription Labeling Among Seniors," *Gerontology* 48, no. 1 (2002): 44–51.

7. C. M. Ruland, "Improving Patient Outcomes by Including Patient Preferences in Nursing Care," *Procedures of the AMIA Symposium* (1998): 448–52; M. Heisler and others, "The Relative Importance of Physician Communication, Participatory Decision Making, and Patient Understanding in Diabetes Self-Management," *Journal of General Internal Medicine* 17, no. 4 (2002): 243–52; S. H. Kaplan, S. Greenfield, and J. E. Ware, "Assessing the Effects of Physician-Patient Interactions on the Outcomes of Chronic Disease," *Medical Care* 27 (suppl) (1989): S100–27.

8. R. B. Deber, N. Kratschmer, and J. Irvine, "What Role Do Patients Wish to Play in Treatment Decision Making?" *Archives of Internal Medicine* 156, no. 13 (1996): 1414–20; J. Benbassat, D. Pilpel, and M. Tidhar, "Patients' Preferences for Participation in Clinical Decision Making: A Review of Published Surveys," *Behavioral Medicine* 24, no. 2 (1998): 81–88; B. McKinstry, "Do Patients Wish to Be Involved in Decision Making in the Consultation? A Cross Sectional Survey with Video Vignettes," *British Medical Journal* 321 (2000): 867–71.

9. *National Survey on Americans as Health Care Consumers: An Update on the Role of Quality Information* (Menlo Park, Calif.: Kaiser Family Foundation, 2000).

10. C. W. DiGiovanni, L. Kang, and J. Manuel, "Patient Compliance in Avoiding Wrong-Site Surgery," *The Journal of Bone and Joint Surgery (American)* 85 (2003): 815–19.

11. E. B. Larson, "Measuring, Monitoring, and Reducing Medical Harm from a Systems Perspective: A Medical Director's Personal Reflections," *Academic Medicine* 77, no. 10 (2002): 993–1000.

12. C. Foster, *There's Something I Have to Tell You. How to Communicate Difficult News in Tough Situations* (New York: Harmony Books, 1997).

13. C. Laine and F. Davidoff, "Patient-Centered Medicine: A Professional Evolution," *Journal of the American Medical Association* 275 (1996): 152–56.

14. D. G. Safran, "Defining the Future of Primary Care: What Can We Learn from Patients?" *Annals of Internal Medicine* 138, no. 3 (2003):

248–55; D. S. Main and others, "Patient Perspectives on the Doctor of the Future," *Family Medicine* 34, no. 4 (2002): 251–57.

15. Materials are available for download on the Web site of the Agency for Healthcare Research and Quality (www.ahrq.gov).

16. Harborview Medical Center, *Ethnic Medicine Information* [http:www. ethnomed.org/]. Accessed June 2003.

17. C. Chantler and J. Johnson, "Patients Should Receive Copies of Letters and Summaries," *British Medical Journal* 325 (2002): 388–89.

18. Harry Cayton, Director of Patient Experience and Public Involvement, United Kingdom Department of Health, London, England, keynote speech, "Copying Letters to Patients," October 30, 2002 [http://www.doh.gov.uk/patientletters/speech.htm].

19. D. Jelley and T. van Zwanenberg, "Copying GP Referral Letters to Patients: Study of Patients' Views," *British Journal of General Practice* 50 (2000): 657–58.

20. More information about the copying letters to patients initiative can be found on the United Kingdom Department of Health Web site: http://www.doh.gov.uk/patientletters.

21. P. L. Spath, "Sharing the Knowledge," *Health Forum Journal* 46, no. 2 (2003): 16–19, 47.

22. M. R. Chassin and E. C. Becher, "The Wrong Patient: Quality Grand Rounds," *Annals of Internal Medicine* 136, no. 11 (2002): 826–33.

23. *Marcus Welby, M.D.: U.S. Medical Drama,* The Museum of Broadcast Communications [http://www.museum.tv]. Accessed June 2003.

24. J. Turow, *Playing Doctor: Television, Storytelling, and Medical Power* (New York: Oxford University Press, 1989).

5

Enabling Patient Involvement
without Increasing Liability Risks

James W. Saxton, Esquire,
and Maggie M. Finkelstein, Esquire

Before coming to the hospital tomorrow morning, use this pen to mark "No" on the knee that I won't be operating on and "Yes" on the knee I will be operating on. That way we'll be sure to operate on the knee that's giving you problems.

Please help remind us to wash our hands before we perform any hands-on procedures. We don't want to spread infections, and hand washing is an important preventive measure.

If at any time during your hospital stay you don't feel safe or have a concern about the care you are receiving, here is the phone number of a person whom you or your family can contact.

Physicians, nurses, and other caregivers are reaching out to patients to encourage them to become active participants in the health care experience. The advancement of safer health care services can be accomplished in part by patients' involvement in their own care and effective collaboration with caregivers. Requesting that patients notify the physician or staff members of perceived mistakes or unsafe situations could ultimately lead to a reduction of adverse events.[1] An example of engaging the patient in error reduction is in the prevention of wrong-site surgery. The patient (or a family member) can be actively involved in the surgery site identification process. There are many other health care situations in which the patient may be able to recognize and prevent errors from occurring.

Regrettably, patients are often an untapped resource when it comes to safeguarding health care services. Several factors affect this state of affairs, perhaps the most pervasive one being the traditional "lone hero" model of the medical profession that can limit the openness and equality of caregiver-patient interactions.[2] This traditional model conflicts with the contemporary values of many patients who are seeking a more collaborative and partnering relationship with practitioners. Physicians and other caregivers must learn how to create legitimate opportunities for patients to be involved in making health care safer and to give them the tools (i.e., knowledge and skills) to be effective safety partners. Numerous suggestions on how this can be accomplished are found throughout this book.

Disclosure and Information Sharing

Practicing true patient involvement and improving communication between patients on the one hand and physicians, nurses, and other caregivers on the other have numerous beneficial effects. They increase patient satisfaction and strengthen mutual trust. Open lines of communication can also help keep patients' expectations in line with reality. All of these benefits can lead to a decrease in professional liability lawsuits as well as a decrease in medical errors.[3] Yet a health care professional's fear of a lawsuit may actually create barriers to effective practitioner-patient partnerships. To solicit patient involvement in error prevention, health care professionals must acknowledge that mistakes can and do happen. Such an admission can be problematic.

A recent study of physicians' attitudes about disclosing actual medical errors suggests that doctors are clearly worried that admitting mistakes can make a lawsuit more likely.[4] This attitude can also inhibit physicians and other caregivers from suggesting to patients that a mistake might happen. Even though studies have repeatedly shown that most medical errors are caused by faulty systems, not people, it is common for practitioners to view mistakes as personal failures.[5] Operating from this belief, it is reasonable for caregivers to deduce that they will be held personally liable should a mistake actually happen. Thus, physicians and other caregivers may be reluctant to engage patients as partners in preventing errors if such interactions are thought to increase the risk of liability lawsuits.

Even though the threat of lawsuits can never be totally eliminated, many of the liability fears associated with frank and complete practitioner-patient dialogue are overstated. By communicating more effectively with patients, practitioners can enhance a patient's health care. Open, honest, and compassionate interactions can help patients understand that they are an important part of the health care team—one in which all team members are trying their best to achieve the best outcomes.

Most medical errors do not occur because of incompetent or reckless people, substandard care, malpractice, or even deliberate mistakes; errors may occur even when the medical care is optimal. Health care is a complex sociotechnological industry and, as with other complex industries, possesses a high potential for error.[6] It would be unfortunate if the fear of personal liability lawsuits holds health care professionals back from enlisting help from patients (and their family members) in error prevention. Another "set of eyes" should be a welcome safeguard in the health care system.

In November 1999, the National Academy of Science's Institute of Medicine released a controversial report that purported to show, for the first time, the extent to which medical errors may cause preventable deaths in the United States. The report estimated that between 44,000 and 98,000 Americans die each year because of medical errors.[7] Even though medical errors may rank as the eighth leading cause of death, true patient collaboration has the potential for improving the detection and prevention of such errors. At the same time, legal issues appear to inhibit effective practitioner-patient partnerships. A better understanding of these legal issues can help physicians, nurses, and other caregivers put to rest some of their fears. Even legal barriers that are both real and significant are not insurmountable. Practitioners can provide a patient with information about his or her own care, including the potential for errors and adverse outcomes, without an increased risk of a lawsuit. Research data have shown that disclosure reduces both the frequency and severity of claims.[8]

Within the context of this chapter, the term *disclosure* is used to describe communications in which the practitioner reveals medical errors, complications, or near misses that occur after the fact, as well as any other practitioner-patient communications about that patient's medical treatment. Practitioner partnering with a patient applies to informed consent discussions on the risks of treatment as well as general information sharing. We don't suggest that the legal standard for informed consent be changed, only that the information-sharing process be enhanced to achieve possible safety benefits for the patient and the caregiver. Throughout this chapter, the terms *disclosure* and *information sharing* are used synonymously. The disclosure or sharing of medical information with patients, however, has cultural, legal, and regulatory implications and considerations.

Culturally, a significant change is needed in our approach to sharing information with patients and their families. Not only does there exist a lack of incentive to disclose relevant information prior to treatment, but health care providers also cite many reasons for an unwillingness to disclose medical errors after they occur. One study in 2000 revealed that physicians were not eager to acknowledge or discuss medical errors for various reasons, including threats of medical malpractice lawsuits, concerns about personal reputation and job security, and the potential for punitive actions by licensing boards.[9]

Clearly, physicians, staff members, and risk managers have been concerned about disclosure of medical errors and its legal implications, but given the current professional liability landscape, disclosure can be a very positive risk reduction measure. Why? Because failure to disclose is now being used by plaintiffs as a basis for the imposition of punitive damages and large verdict awards. When information sharing is done right—the right way, at the right time, by the right people—the potential for litigation and large verdicts can be reduced.

The legal questions related to disclosure fall into two categories: information sharing about the potential for medical errors (preintervention) and information sharing following the occurrence of an incident or medical error (postintervention). Following is a discussion of the liability fears that accompany disclosure in these two categories, together with recommendations for how these fears can be confronted, minimized, or even eliminated.

Preintervention Communication

The pursuit of safer health care services can be advanced by patients' involvement in their own care, better communication between practitioners and patients, and inclusion of patients as partners on the health care team. The effects of practicing true patient involvement and increasing practitioner-patient communication are beneficial in many ways. They increase patient satisfaction and strengthen the bond between the clinician and the patient. As a result, patients are more likely to follow the recommended course of treatment. Open lines of communication also keep patients' expectations in line with reality. All of these benefits lead to a decrease in professional liability lawsuits as well as a decrease in medical errors.[10] There are two aspects of preintervention communication: general information sharing and the informed consent process.

Patients may be in the best position to watch for medical errors, and for this reason patients may be one of our most underutilized safety resources. The patient has the personal incentive for a positive outcome and may be the most aware of his or her health and the needs associated with treatment. It only makes sense then for practitioners to partner with patients. Some of the measures intended to reinforce the practitioner-patient relationship as a team effort include the following:

- Developing a physician-patient agreement that provides a brief explanation of the health care process and its complexities
- Requesting that patients notify physicians or staff members of any treatment mistakes or errors
- Encouraging patients to be more accountable for their own health[11]

Another useful patient-practitioner collaboration tool that is gaining popularity is a patient journal. In a patient journal all the important information necessary for compliance and monitoring of a patient's care is kept in one place. A journal would be particularly useful in obstetrics, where compliance and self-monitoring by the patient is particularly important. However, the concept could be used in any area of care where the health care providers are counting on the patients to not only monitor their own care but to also actively participate. A journal can be a very specific educational tool for patients and their families to positively encourage participation. A portion of the journal could include a section on safety issues so that patients and their families are encouraged to be vigilant in recognizing and preventing mistakes.

In March 2002, the Joint Commission on Accreditation of Healthcare Organizations partnered with the Centers for Medicare and Medicaid Services to launch a national campaign called "Speak Up." The campaign is intended to encourage patients to become actively involved in their own health care. In response, hospitals around the country are encouraging patients to do the following:

1. Ask questions about their own care
2. Make sure they are receiving the proper treatment
3. Educate themselves
4. Know what medications they take
5. Participate in their own health care treatment decisions

Figure 5-1 lists some of the safety suggestions offered to patients and families on the Web site of Lowell General Hospital, Lowell, Massachusetts.[12]

These types of communications are examples of health care providers pursuing active participation of patients as members of a health care team. It brings expectations more in line with reality at the same time it informs the patient about potential mistakes and irregularities that do and can exist. And while it makes the patient more vigilant, the health care provider must be cognizant that such partnering needs to be done in the right way—it is important to

Figure 5-1.   Safety Information Disclosed to Patients on the Web Site of Lowell General Hospital

Your Role in Patient Safety

These are ways you can help us give you the best care:

- Speak up if you have questions or concerns about your care.
- If you don't understand something, ask! It's your body and you have a right to know.
- Tell your doctor or nurse if something doesn't seem quite right.
- Expect health care workers to introduce themselves when they enter your room and look for their identification badge.
- Tell the health care worker right away if you think he or she has confused you with another patient.
- Know what medicines you take and why you take them.
- Know what time of day you normally receive a medication. If it doesn't happen, ask your nurse or doctor why you didn't get your medicine.
- If you do not recognize a medication, be sure that it is for you.
- Make sure your nurse or doctor knows who you are, that is, checks your wristband or asks your name before he or she gives any medication or treatment.
- Be involved in all decisions about your treatment—you are part of the health care team.
- You might want to ask a trusted family member or friend to help you. They can help remember answers to questions and speak up for you if you cannot.
- Write down important facts your doctor tells you, so that you can look for more information later. And ask your doctor or nurse if he or she has any written information you can keep.
- Ask your doctor the purpose of any new test or medication.
- Read all medical forms and make sure you understand them before you sign anything. If you don't understand, ask your doctor or nurse to explain them.

Patient Rights and Responsibilities

As a patient at Lowell General Hospital, you are the primary member of your health care team and have the right and responsibility to participate to ensure the safe delivery of care. You may request copies of hospital policies and procedures or practices that relate to care, treatment and responsibility.

Patient Advocate
Lowell General Hospital
978-937-6458

Source: Lowell General Hospital, Lowell, Massachusetts. See the full text of the site at http://www.lowellgeneral.org/features/patient/whilehere.asp?open=1# YourRoleinPatientSafe. Reprinted with permission.

put certain statements in the correct context. For example, while partnering with a patient to prevent wrong-site surgery, the physician and staff members should explain that wrong-site surgery occurs only infrequently. In a recent study on the incidence of wrong-site surgery among hand surgeons, it was reported that such errors occur once in every 27,686 procedures.[13]

Family-Centered Care

True patient involvement and partnering with patients can have beneficial effects on a patient's health. One particularly innovative movement is the advocacy of family-centered care. Dr. Nicholas Masi, director of family-centered care at the Joe DiMaggio Children's Hospital, Fort Lauderdale, Florida, and former practicing psychologist, is helping to create opportunities for patient and family involvement in health services.[14] In an interview with the authors, Dr. Masi explained that obstetrics was one of the first services to embrace family-centered care; however, patient demand has expanded this model of care to other services, such as pediatrics. Dr. Masi would like to see family-centered care as the norm, not only in children's health care facilities, but also in adult care areas as well.

According to Dr. Masi, family-centered care is a different way of providing patient treatment, and effecting this change requires a cultural change in the mind-set of health care providers. At the Joe DiMaggio Children's Hospital, for example, family members are to be viewed as caregivers, not visitors; the health care practitioners are the people considered to be visitors. To support this cultural change, the organization is working on a language change to be used by staff and to be evidenced in job descriptions and other facility documents.

Dr. Masi is also encouraging physicians to include family members on patient rounds. He finds that when families are involved in their child's care, for example, several positive outcomes occur, including the following:

- The child's rate of return to the hospital for significant complications is reduced.

- The parent-child bond is enhanced.
- The child's risk of an incident involving social or developmental issues goes down.
- Families are better able to cope with their child's illness.

Positive outcomes have been particularly evident in the neonatal unit. The hospital has designed a room, somewhat like a hotel room, where parents may stay overnight to take care of their infant when discharge is imminent. This allows the parents to become comfortable with caring for their child before going home. Any issues that arise are discussed and remedied while the child is still hospitalized.

Informed Consent

Because an essential patient safety tool is communication, it is vital for physicians and other caregivers to establish open lines of communication with patients. Communication establishes trust and provides a framework for discussion between the caregiver and the patient that is essential to the success of information sharing. One of the first instances in which open communication is beneficial is during the informed consent process—disclosure preintervention. The informed consent process is a patient-specific form of communication, not just a form that must be completed and signed. Although the legal principles of informed consent vary from state to state, the general principles are the same.

- The proposed treatment/procedure is explained.
- The known risks and alternatives to the proposed treatment/procedure are disclosed.
- The risks of not undergoing any treatment/procedure are discussed.

The informed consent process is an opportunity for the patient to ask questions and receive answers, as well as an opportunity for the physician to obtain patient-specific information so that the appropriate course of treatment for the patient can be recommended. A properly executed informed consent opens dialogue and involves the patient in his or her own care. As a result, the patient feels cared for, listened to, and respected.[15] In addition, the informed consent process allows the patient to make a truly informed decision. As a result, should the patient actually incur one of the risks, it is no longer an "unexpected" result. Accordingly, the patient's expectations remain in line with reality.[16] Otherwise, patients become suspicious, as well as angered, when they hear for the first time about a potential complication after it occurs.[17]

Through the informed consent process, physicians are already disclosing possible medical errors, which may be "packaged" as potential risks during the process. On the other hand, many of the errors caused by breakdowns in the systems of care would not be typically referred to as risks. For example, such incidents as wrong-site surgery, an infection caused by a break in sterile technique, or medication errors are not specifically explained during the informed consent process. However, a discussion of the potential for these mishaps could be part of the preintervention communication. Although at first blush it may appear awkward for physicians or other caregivers to point out the potential for mistakes, it is likely that patients will welcome such discussions. Studies suggest, in fact, that many patients are seeking more personal control of their health care experience.

With that said, it is important to strike a balance between the art of reassurance and information sharing. Even though information sharing builds the confidence of a patient through partnering, it is essential to also consider when too much information may actually harm the patient and/or the care of the patient. An increased vigilance by the patient is important for his or her own safety, but it is also important that health care providers don't go overboard to the point where the disclosure of potential medical errors actually acts to alarm an already anxious patient. In addition, there is a point at which qualitative information becomes denuded and thus stripped of meaning, preventing a patient from focusing on the essential aspects of his or her care. Further, physicians and their staff often operate under strict time constraints, and for this reason health care providers may be unable to disclose every potential risk no matter its likelihood of occurrence. These are only challenges to be faced, however, and should not be seen as obstacles.

The informed consent process can be a valuable patient safety tool when used as a true patient education process in which medical risks as well as potential safety issues are disclosed.[18] At first, practitioners may think discussions of safety issues will lead to greater patient anxiety or mistrust of caregivers, thinking that has contributed to our present state of affairs. In reality, patients want to know and want to help. It is clear that patients expect to be kept informed and involved throughout their treatment. A participant in a recent study of patient perspectives on the ideal physician commented: "I would like to be informed about what's going on. It's probably the most critical thing in having good health care. . . . Treat me like I'm human and intelligent."[19] The information provided during the informed consent process, both risks and alternatives as well as safety issues, is the type of information that could be contained in a patient journal.

Disclosing the Potential for Error

In the future, will a physician or other health care provider have an affirmative obligation to disclose potential safety issues and then be liable for failing to do so after a medical error actually comes to fruition? As more information about the incidence of medical errors comes to light, does it become a standard of care to disclose the potential for errors? At this time, it would appear unlikely that such disclosures will become standard practice. The legal analysis for such potential claims follows.

If the potential for well-known medical errors is required to be disclosed as part of the informed consent process, does a failure to disclose result in a lost opportunity for the patient to guard against the potential error? Such a claim would have to be alleged under a negligence theory and would need to be linked causally to any injury that occurred. Or is it simply that a discussion on the potential error should have been part of the informed consent process?

As we know, some potential errors are already being included in informed consent discussions, such as the potential for an infection. At the present time, however, informed consent requirements in most jurisdictions don't embrace other types of systemwide errors or remote risks, like wrong-site surgery. Notwithstanding the above, the discussion of medical errors could reduce the potential for a lawsuit in the first place. The patient would no longer be surprised when a mistake occurs, making postintervention disclosure less contentious.

Information sharing with a patient preintervention is a valuable tool that enhances a patient's health care experience. Involving patients in their own care leads to better outcomes and provides a framework for preintervention discussions. Of course, the informed consent stage is essential for disclosing the potential for material risks, but it is also a time to begin the process of involving patients more actively in their own care. Information sharing, including informed consent, helps to keep patients' expectations in line with reality. Once the provider-patient communication lines have been opened, the positive aspects of this collaboration can carry over into postintervention interactions. And it is at the post-intervention point that many liability fears are realized, but those fears can—and should be—overcome.

Postintervention Communication

Full disclosure of a medical error after it has occurred has many potential advantages, including reduction of the severity and frequency of claims. Often, however, health care providers assume just the opposite—that disclosure of a medical error will result in a deterioration of the provider-patient relationship or influence the patient to seek legal action. Following are several specific concerns related to disclosure of a mistake:

- Liability implications
- Lawsuits
- Liability insurance coverage

- Reimbursement
- Peer review proceedings

A discussion of these and several related points follows.

Liability Implications

Health care organizations and physicians often fear that disclosing a medical error to the patient or family will be perceived as an admission of liability. Will the disclosure be used against the facility or the practitioner at trial? In answering this question, it is important to understand that disclosure of an error, done in the right fashion, does not mean that the facility or practitioner was negligent. There is often a misperception by the medical community as to what constitutes legal negligence.

Legal Negligence

The legal standard of negligence requires that a plaintiff prove, to a reasonable degree of medical certainty, that the conduct of a physician or other caregiver breached the applicable "standard of care" and that the breach in the care legally caused the plaintiff's injuries. As to a professional physician, the standard of care generally requires that a physician have and use the same knowledge and skill and exercise the same care as that which is usually possessed and exercised in the medical profession. A specialist must generally meet a higher standard of care: a specialist must have and use the same knowledge and skill and exercise the same care as that possessed and exercised by others in the same specialty. A physician or specialist who fails to meet the applicable standard is considered negligent.

Meanwhile, a hospital or physician's practice can be held legally liable for the negligent actions of its physicians and staff (including nurses) under an agency theory as long as a causative connection to the damage is established as well. In addition, some states have extended the doctrine of corporate negligence to hospitals, finding that hospitals owe a direct duty of care to patients cared for in their facilities.

Case law in many jurisdictions establishes that an error in judgment is not negligence. A distinction is made between actual malpractice, an error in judgment, and sources of adverse outcomes that are not the fault of the physician. These legal distinctions can become blurred and, hence, a source of confusion. A physician, hospital, or other health care provider is *legally* negligent only when the care rendered by the physician (or hospital in the case of corporate negligence) breached the standard of care (explained above). Further, even if a health care provider has breached the standard of care, the health care provider can be liable to the plaintiff only if the plaintiff further shows that the breach in care *legally* caused the injuries complained of by the plaintiff (that is, generally, that the actions of the health care provider were a substantial factor in bringing about the harm incurred by the plaintiff).[20] If no such connection is made between the actions of the health care provider and the injuries incurred by the plaintiff, the health care provider is not liable for the injuries sustained by the plaintiff. In other words, as long as we are thoughtful in the way disclosure occurs, it will not be used as a judicial admission, and a plaintiff must still establish how that breach was the legal cause of the injury before liability will attach.

Statute of Limitations

Failing to disclose a medical error in a timely manner may potentially influence the statute of limitations (the period given to a potential plaintiff for filing suit). If a defendant is found to have concealed a medical error, whether actively or unintentionally, under certain circumstances such concealment may act to extend the time for filing of a professional liability lawsuit.[21]

Let us consider a situation in which a state law provides that a claimant has two years from the date of injury to file a professional liability claim and a physician has actively concealed an error in a surgery for an ulcer. Unknown to the patient, the sponge count was off, and the physician and staff were unable to locate the missing sponge. Subsequently, the patient incurred abdominal pain of unknown etiology. Five years after the ulcer surgery, during exploratory surgery in attempts to discover the source of abdominal pain, a sponge was discovered. By failing to disclose the error in sponge count, the patient had no reason to know the source of the pain could be from a retained sponge. Instead of the patient's being required to file a lawsuit within two years of the first surgery, a legal principle—the "discovery rule"—could allow a plaintiff to file a lawsuit within two years of the discovery of the retained sponge, which occurred during the second surgery (five years later). Under the discovery rule, the limitation statute in malpractice cases does not start to run (i.e., the cause of action does not accrue) until the date of the discovery of the malpractice, or the date when, by the exercise of reasonable care and diligence, the patient should have discovered the wrongful act (*Black's Law Dictionary*, 6th ed.).

In the above example, concealment of an error extended the statute of limitations by five years. This is a significant length of time that could have an effect on the ability to secure accurate data, records, witnesses, and recollections in defense of the malpractice action. This example, in which an error was concealed, is not to be confused with the so-called discovery rule that extends the statute of limitations when a patient, even though he or she is diligent, could have "discovered" the relationship between the care and injury. This situation is confronted most often in misdiagnosis of cancer cases.

Research by DecisionQuest, Inc., a nationwide trial and jury consulting firm, has shown that jurors expect disclosure of medical errors to occur whether it results in injury to the patient or not. This research finding is not unexpected because jurors are very much like the average patient. When asked about disclosure preferences, patients reportedly want even minor errors to be revealed to them by their physician.[22] These findings suggest that disclosure of medical mistakes may actually work in favor of the physician and the provider facility. Otherwise, jurors may perceive a cover-up and conjure up conspiracy theories and reasons that the physician or hospital is "hiding" something.

DecisionQuest advocates that the defense team consider early on how to use the communication of disclosure to its advantage.

The authors have been involved in effectuating policies whereby disclosure has been used to effectively diffuse the patient's and family's emotions after an adverse event resulting in a move to a fast-track claims process when appropriate. It is necessary for health care providers to be educated about such types of policies, which take time and other resources to effectively develop and to train health care providers.

Apologies

It has been argued that health care providers would feel more at ease in apologizing for a medical error if such apologies were prohibited from being admitted as evidence at a trial.[23] The state of California enacted such a statute in 2000, joining at least two other states with similar statutes.[24] It has been suggested that such laws could reduce medical errors as well as lawsuits. In the well-regarded study by Hickson and others, it was discovered that nearly one-quarter of all professional liability suits (prenatal suits) were filed because a patient was angered that the health care provider had not been honest or had misled the patient.[25] Even if an apology doesn't prevent a lawsuit, it may at least decrease animosity and lead to a quicker resolution of the case.[26] Apologies can be useful, but they should be made during an expression of empathy, not as an admission of fault. This is another area where training and education of health care providers and risk managers can make a real difference.

Multiple Defendants

Disclosure of a mistake can be problematic when other potential defendants may be involved with the error or complication. Consider an incident that occurs when a surgeon, anesthesiologist, medical specialist, and nurses are all actively involved in caring for a patient. The disclosure process must be coordinated because each provider may be a potential defendant. Questions to be addressed include: Who will speak on behalf of all involved parties at meetings with patients and/or families? What will be said and when? Each party, of course, will be wary of where blame or fault may be unintentionally placed. The logistics can become complicated but should not be an excuse for failing to disclose the facts and circumstances of an incident with the patient and/or the patient's family. As has been discussed, failure to disclose has more significant adverse affects than does disclosure to *all* involved. Working through the logistics and concerns is warranted and is being successfully accomplished throughout the country.

Litigation Implications

Health care professionals fear that disclosure will prompt professional liability lawsuits, as evidenced by the fact that fear of medical malpractice litigation has been cited as the most common barrier for developing and implementing disclosure policies.[27] However, from a liability standpoint there is growing support that information sharing is an aid to the doctor or hospital.

Early evidence suggests that disclosure does not result in an increase in lawsuits. For example, consider the Veterans Administration (VA) Medical Center in Lexington, Kentucky. In the 1980s, it suffered two large awards in medical malpractice cases (totaling more than $1.5 million). In 1987, the medical center adopted a disclosure policy and procedure, which involves full disclosure to the patient and/or family of a medical error that has caused injury. The disclosure includes an apology and a discussion of compensation and liability. Although the policy has resulted in some settlements where no litigation may have been instituted had the disclosure not been made, to date full disclosure has not resulted in higher liability payments.[28]

One study found that the economic benefit of disclosure is positive, resulting in reasonable settlements and fair compensation to the injured parties.[29] One of the researchers, Steve S. Kraman, pulmonologist and hospital chief of staff at the VA Medical Center in Lexington, stated that although the total number of litigation cases increased following implementation of the full disclosure policy, the cost per case decreased dramatically.[30] On average, the medical center makes 14 payments per year (which is a high number for a veterans hospital), but the average payment per case is only $15,000, compared with the average payment at other VA hospitals of $100,000. The cost savings here may be due largely to the lack of full-fledged litigation, which is far more expensive.[31]

The effectiveness of the Lexington facility's disclosure policy led to implementation of a similar policy throughout all Veterans Health Administration facilities in 1995.[32] The policy requires that the medical center do the following:

- Inform the patient and/or his or her family of an event.

- Assure the patient and/or his or her family that medical measures have been implemented.

- Disclose steps that are being taken to minimize further personal or financial loss.

- Advise the patient and/or his or her family of the procedures for recovering compensation for the harm.

Can this same policy of disclosure work well in the private sector? The Veterans Health Administration system is somewhat different from a legal standpoint. Doctors working in the system are protected from personal liability and cannot be individually named in a malpractice suit.[33] Medical malpractice lawsuits brought against a federal facility must be filed under the Federal Tort Claims Act, which bars punitive damages.[34] In addition, if a patient's injuries are service related, he or she may qualify for financial assistance. In contrast, a physician operating in the private sector may be sued personally.[35] However, in both instances, any financial payment made on behalf of the physician must be reported to the National Practitioner's Data Bank.[36]

Despite these factors, there is no reason why similar disclosure policies implemented in the private sector would not yield the same results as those that are being seen within the Veterans Health Administration. As yet, no similar studies have been performed in the private sector, but it is clear that the same principles of open and honest communication, early disclosure, and coordinated efforts can reduce the severity of claims. The substantive area of law is governed by state malpractice laws in both cases, so no legal barriers would prohibit such a system in the private sector. By implementing a system similar to that in the VA system, private sector organizations really would be implementing a risk management program that could similarly lead to reasonable settlements and just compensation to injured parties.

Although preliminary results suggest that full disclosure of medical errors can reduce liability risks, fear of the potential for litigation continues to be a significant barrier to open and honest provider-patient communication.[37] This fear is most likely derived from the inherent nature of tort law: its perceived intent is to punish and deter future conduct by both the wrongdoer and others who might act similarly in the future. However, this perception is not legally accurate except when punitive damages are asserted; and punitive damages are claimed when a health care provider's actions are intentional or reckless.[38] This barrier to full disclosure is one that could be alleviated by the right tort reform measures. In addition, it is important that the physician or individual disclosing the medical error do it properly to prevent the appearance of an admission of liability and not discuss fault or blame. Keep in mind as well that it is both the *frequency* and the *severity* of claims that health care providers are seeking to reduce.

Effect on Reputation

Another barrier to full disclosure of medical errors is the fear that sharing information will lead to adverse publicity for the physician and/or the facility. Adverse publicity would affect a physician personally as well as the reputation of his or her practice, which, of course, would have a negative financial impact for the physician. For hospitals and other provider organizations, adverse publicity can lessen the community's trust and confidence in the facility and its staff members and ultimately affect market share.

Does the fear of loss of reputation make health care providers reluctant to disclose information about a medical error? In a study by Lamb and others, it was found that the threat of negative news media coverage did not influence a hospital's willingness to disclose information to any of its patients.[39] In fact, proper disclosure prevents misinformation and reduces the public's perception that the hospital is hiding something. Reinforcing the value of open and honest communication with patients is Hickson's study of perinatal injury lawsuits—50 percent of the lawsuits were motivated by suspicions of a cover-up.[40] If the media do request information about an adverse event, it is essential that physicians and hospitals get expert assistance from professionals in risk management and public relations and also consider patient confidentiality issues.

Liability Coverage Implications

Contracts for insurance may inadvertently inhibit disclosure reform efforts.[41] Disclosure may violate the contract of professional liability insurance between the physician and the insurance carrier and thus threaten insurance coverage for any claims related to the disclosure. Generally, physicians are prohibited by contract from hindering the defense of a claim, and some professional liability carriers require consent from the insurance carrier before the physician may apologize or admit liability. The insurance carrier may construe an apology or any other disclosure as an admission of liability, thereby violating the insurance contract, and such a violation may allow the insurance carrier to deny coverage. Thus, many of the current contracts for liability insurance could be a disincentive to disclosure. The same is true for professional liability coverage maintained by a hospital or other health care organization, whether coverage is for the entity itself or maintained by the entity on behalf of its employees, including physicians and nurses.

Kraman maintains that professional liability insurers are often interested in small payouts, and for this reason insurers would have to be convinced of the economic benefit of disclosure, especially full disclosure like that implemented in the Veterans Health Administration.[42] However, this contract-related disincentive is likely to disappear as more insurance carriers become enlightened and actually encourage disclosure for obvious reasons—it *reduces* the potential for both frequency and severity of claims when done appropriately. More recently, enlightened professional liability insurers have begun to move to the forefront of encouraging appropriate, coordinated disclosure and should continue to educate and train accordingly.

Peer Review Implications

Concerns specific to health care professionals involve peer review, credentialing, and licensure. Physicians and other licensed professionals may fear that disclosing a medical error would trigger peer review, sanctions, or a licensing review by a state board. For example, if a physician has documented the disclosure of several medical errors, would that situation prompt a peer review, disciplinary proceedings, or a licensing review? Such investigations would be counterproductive unless the reason for the error could truly be associated with individual competency problems.

To alleviate fears that disclosures will prompt peer review or disciplinary proceedings, it is recommended that disclosure policies and procedures make it clear that sharing information about a medical error with the patient (or patient's family) is not an admission of responsibility for purposes of peer review, sanctioning, and reporting requirements.[43] This clarification could alleviate some concerns about disclosure for physicians and other health care professionals.

Achieving Full Disclosure

The legal and cultural obstacles to full disclosure of medical errors need to be overcome so that patients (and their families) can be truly engaged as partners in the health care experience. Even though the legal concerns and fears are real, all stakeholders in this issue can have their agendas advanced by a system that embraces postintervention disclosure. The issues are complex and the solutions will take time and investments in change. To create a culture of safety, senior leaders and management must commit to changing the status quo and convey that commitment to physicians and staff members. Many organizations start the cultural change process by developing and disseminating a policy on patient and family member communication following an error or near miss.[44] The key issues surrounding disclosure are summarized in figure 5-2.

Figure 5-2.   Summary of Issues Related to Postintervention Disclosure

- Explain to the patient and/or family members that an *unexpected* error has occurred (never speculate).
- Inform them that an investigation is going to occur or has begun.
- Apologize to the patient and/or family members.
- Assure the patient and/or family members that the problem will be fixed so that the error will not occur again.
- Select the appropriate communicator.
- Involve risk management professionals.
- Assure the patient and/or family members that the patient's personal safety is of foremost importance and describe what is being done to safeguard it.
- Don't place blame or fault.
- Provide the patient and/or family members with contact information so that they can obtain further information.
- Document the disclosure—where, when, and who was in attendance—in the patient's medical chart.
- Document specifics of the disclosure in risk management files.
- Be mindful of confidentiality implications.

Effective patient communication needs to be incorporated into the culture of safety to promote disclosure. Recall that failed communication is often the "major instigating factor in lawsuits."[45] Patients (or their families) often file suits just to learn about the facts of what happened. Recall as well the many benefits of better provider-patient communication: a framework for discussion, patient involvement, patients feeling like partners in their own care, improved health of the patient, and a decrease in the potential number of professional liability lawsuits. Nonetheless, postintervention communication should be accomplished with certain parameters in mind. After the occurrence of a medical error, patients want three things.

- An explanation of what happened
- An apology
- An assurance that the cause will be fixed so that the error will not occur again[46]

The doctor may be the most logical communicator for disclosing an error to a patient, even when the mistake was caused by a system problem that may have been out of the physician's control. Ideally, the physician has already established an open line of communication with the patient as well as a rapport. Of course, there will be times when it is impossible for the physician to conduct the discussion, or times when a particular physician is just not capable of properly conducting such a discussion. For this reason, the organization should designate a properly trained backup individual. Further, even if it is the doctor communicating the error, the process should be a collaborative effort with professional risk managers and, when appropriate, legal counsel.

It is never appropriate for the physician and/or hospital to remain silent following a harmful incident, as this approach is often perceived as a cover-up by the patient or family. For documentation and verification purposes, a second individual should be in attendance during the disclosure—risk management personnel or another individual designated by the facility.

When multiple practitioners are involved, coordinate the disclosure process so that everyone's rights are protected and a unified message delivered. The attendance of certain individuals during a discussion should always be coordinated with risk management professionals and the appropriate professional liability insurer.

The information disclosed to the patient and/or the family should be limited to what is actually known. Never speculate. In many instances, it is impossible to know immediately exactly what went wrong, but the disclosure conversation needs to take place as soon as possible after an incident, so don't wait until the investigation results are known. The patient and/or family need to be told how and/or why the incident occurred and that the cause may not be known until a later time. It is important to let the patient and family know that an investigation will be taking place and the time when further discussions may occur. The main concern should be the patient's safety and well-being. The patient must be given the information necessary for understanding how his or her continued treatment will be affected by the incident and needs to feel continued involvement in the health care experience. Disclosure is not a time to blame or place fault.

Specifically, acknowledge that an *unexpected* error has occurred, where, when, and the circumstances of the incident. Disclose the consequences of the error to continued treatment and who will be managing the patient's care from then on. Take time to answer questions posed by the patient and family. Be regretful if necessary, and apologize for what has occurred (not to be confused with an apology for any kind of negligent actions). Empathize with the patient and family and provide information on support services if necessary.

Explain who has been informed of the error, the investigation and review that will take place, and steps that will be taken so the same error will not happen in the future. Let the patient and family know that as more information becomes available, they will be informed. In the meantime, provide them with contact information so that any questions that arise in the future can be answered.

Involve risk management personnel as well as liability insurers from an informational point of view. Risk management professionals can provide valuable insight into disclosure practices and assist in coordinating messages. Document the disclosure and any subsequent conversations in your investigative peer review file. In the patient's medical records, it should only be noted that a conversation took place, when, where, and who was in attendance. All further details, including what was discussed, that the family and/or patient had the opportunity to ask questions, and that assistance was offered, should be documented in risk management files. Failure to document the disclosure may lead jurors to believe that the conversation never took place. In addition, some states require mandatory disclosure of certain medical errors. In such cases, a letter such as the one shown in figure 5-3 must be sent to the patient.

There are rare circumstances when it may be necessary to withhold information from a patient and/or family. On occasion, the potential harm to a patient's health will outweigh the benefit of disclosure, or there may even be psychological reasons for withholding information. In these instances, document the reasons for

Figure 5-3. **Sample Letter to Patient for Medical Error Disclosure Documentation**

Date: _____

Dear _____,

ABC Hospital is committed to providing quality medical care for its patients and the communities it serves. Despite constant and committed efforts to provide and improve patient care, medical errors sometimes unfortunately occur.

Please do not misconstrue this notification as an admission of liability but rather as ABC Hospital's long-standing commitment to respect the rights of patients and their families to be informed about the occurrence of serious events, and to analyze such events to improve patient care and prevent recurrence of such events. This notification confirms our discussion with you concerning the occurrence of a serious event and the steps that *[we are taking] [were taken]* to remedy the problem.

On *[date of event]* a medical error occurred involving *[patient name]*.

On *[date of notification]* at *[time of notification]*, a meeting was held with *[names of those in attendance]*.

As we discussed, *[details of the event]*.

We strongly encourage you to call *[name of risk manager or patient safety officer]* at *[phone number]* if any further questions or concerns arise. Your continued satisfaction with the care *[you/your family member]* receive[s] at ABC Hospital is our primary goal, and we would appreciate any other questions or comments that you may have regarding this matter.

_____

[Printed name of staff who provided notification]

_____

[Signature of staff who provided notification]

_____

Note: This example meets the requirements of some state laws for the disclosure of medical errors to patients. Consult legal counsel for the requirements for such disclosure in your jurisdiction.

Source: James W. Saxton, Esquire, Stevens & Lee, Lancaster, Pennsylvania.

withholding the information. Put generic information regarding the circumstances in the patient's chart, but set forth the specific reasons for withholding information in the risk management file.

Of course, if it is suspected that a patient's death was caused by a medical error, it makes this process even more important. It is necessary for the process of disclosure in such a situation to be handled in a timely manner. Otherwise, the same principles discussed above apply.

Once the disclosure process has been initiated, what is most important is that caregivers learn from the error. Although there is often a desire to quickly move beyond an unpleasant situation, it is critical to conduct a complete analysis of what happened and why. In other words, there are two important obligations when a medical error occurs. First, by properly sharing information about the incident with the patient and/or family, health care professionals will have met their ethical and, at times, legal responsibilities. Full disclosure will reduce the risk of liability claims and minimize the potential for a large and severe judgment award. Second, full disclosure sets the stage for performance improvement by bringing together those involved so that preventive measures can be taken. In essence, the health care providers now possess information on how and why certain medical errors occur, which provide the means for future prevention.

Disclosure and Confidentiality

A component of the provider-patient relationship is confidentiality. Physicians and other health care professionals are generally prohibited from disclosing a patient's medical information to others without the patient's consent,[47] which could prevent the disclosure of medical errors to the patient's family. Recent privacy regulations promulgated by the U.S. Department of Health and Human Services (which are amendments to the Health Care Insurance Portability and Accountability Act, or HIPAA) implicate the disclosure of medical information (and potentially medical errors) to a patient's "family member, other relative, or a close personal friend of the [patient], or any other person identified by the [patient]."[48] The health care provider, however, is permitted to do so only with the consent of the patient; where the patient has had an opportunity to object but fails to do so; or where, based on the exercise of the health care provider's professional judgment, he or she reasonably can infer that the patient does not object to disclosure.[49] If, however, the patient is not present or has not had the opportunity to agree or to object to disclosure because of incapacity or an emergency, the health care provider may disclose information that is directly relevant to the individual's involvement with the patient's care if, under the health care provider's professional judgment, the provider believes that the disclosure is in the best interest of the patient.

Because these national regulations are so new and the language so broad and vague, it is impossible to know how they will be interpreted by the appropriate reviewing entity and under what specific factual scenarios involving disclosure they may apply. But the regulations are a legal concern that health care providers need to be aware of and follow where appropriate. In addition, health care providers should be aware that these regulations specifically provide that if a state statute allows more stringent privacy requirements, then the state law is applicable and needs to be followed.[50] For this reason, health care providers covered by the regulations must understand their particular state's laws regarding confidentiality and privacy of medical information.

Legal Risks versus Patient Safety

When communicated in the right way by the right people at the right time, information sharing and disclosure are beneficial to all participants—the patient and health care providers. For the patient it can lead to better health outcomes. The fears of health care providers about information sharing and disclosure are understandable but need to be overcome and can be accomplished without increasing professional liability exposure. The development of effective policies and the education of health care providers and risk managers is essential to alleviate their fears of the effect of information sharing and disclosure on health care providers' liability, insurance coverage, reimbursement, peer review, credentialing, and licensing. Effective information and disclosure, in fact, can result in a reduction of both the frequency and severity of claims.

Effective preintervention communication establishes a discussion framework that has many benefits, including improved patient-practitioner partnerships and better patient care and outcomes. State laws generally require that a patient be informed of a proposed medical treatment or procedure as well as its risks and alternatives and the risks of not undergoing the treatment or procedure. This process allows a patient to make a truly informed decision and, when done properly, keeps a patient's expectations in line with reality. Preintervention communication is also an opportunity to solidify the patient-practitioner partnership.

Patient partnering is an important aspect of promoting a culture of safety. It allows a patient to be truly involved in his or her own care, which strengthens the caregiver-patient bond and promotes the health of the patient. This in turn can lead to a decrease in the incidence of medical errors and resulting professional liability claims.

If a medical mistake does occur, health care providers face many obstacles that can (but should not) prevent the sharing of information with a patient. These obstacles include liability implications, litigation implications, reputation issues, liability coverage, and peer review ramifications. Even though all of these impediments are real, they are often overstated. Postintervention disclosure done in the right way, as noted previously, can actually lead to a decrease in professional liability lawsuits, because the patient and the family are informed and involved, and confusion and anger are diffused. Further, open disclosure of incidents allows health care professionals to learn from medical errors so that similar occurrences can be prevented in the future. As the VA hospital in Kentucky has found, open and honest communication can lead to a decrease in liability claim payouts and lawsuits.

Being aware of the potential legal, cultural, and regulatory issues in information sharing will promote more effective information sharing and patient involvement. True patient involvement can promote the culture of safety for patients that everyone is looking to achieve. It is time to move the sharing of information with patients to the next level. Although at first it seems counterintuitive, a more informed and educated patient is a safer patient and one whose expectations are more realistic. Many of the perceived legal barriers to pre- and postintervention disclosure can be overcome through education and initiative.

References

1. B. A. Liang, "A System of Medical Error Disclosure," *Quality and Safety in Health Care* 11 (2002): 64–68.
2. G. B. Hickson and others, "Patient Complaints and Malpractice Risk," *Journal of the American Medical Association* 287, no. 22 (2002): 2951–57; M. B. Kapp, "Legal Anxieties and Medical Mistakes," *Journal of General Internal Medicine* 12, no. 12 (1997): 787–88.
3. W. Levinson and others, "Physician-Patient Communication: The Relationship with Malpractice Claims Among Primary Care Physicians and Surgeons," *Journal of the American Medical Association* 227, no. 7 (1999): 553–59.
4. T. H. Gallagher and others, "Patients' and Physicians' Attitudes Regarding the Disclosure of Medical Errors," *Journal of the American Medical Association* 289, no. 8 (2003): 1001–7.
5. M. Ringel, "Mistakes in Medicine," *Nexus* (March/April 2003) [http://www.nexuspub.com/articles/2003/march2003/zen_mar_2003.htm].
6. B. A. Liang, "Error in Medicine: Legal Impediments to U.S. Reform," *Journal of Health Politics, Policy and Law* 24, no. 1 (1999): 27–58.
7. L. T. Kohn, J. M. Corrigan, and M. S. Donaldson, eds., *To Err Is Human: Building a Safer Health System,* Institute of Medicine Committee on Quality of Health Care in America (Washington, D.C.: National Academy Press, 1999).
8. See G. B. Hickson and others, "Factors That Prompted Families to File Medical Malpractice Claims Following Perinatal Injuries," *Journal of the American Medical Association* 267 (1992): 1359–63; C. Vincent, M. Young, and A. Phillips, "Why Do People Sue Doctors? A Study of Patients and Relatives Taking Legal Action," *Lancet* 343 (1994): 1609–13; S. S. Kraman and G. Hamm, "Risk Management: Extreme Honesty May Be the Best Policy," *Annals of Internal Medicine* 131 (1999): 963–67.
9. J. B. Sexton, E. J. Thomas, and R. L. Helmreich, "Error, Stress, and Teamwork in Medicine and Aviation: Cross Sectional Surveys," *British Medical Journal* 320 (2000): 745–49.

10. W. Levinson and others, "Physician-Patient Communication: The Relationship with Malpractice Claims Among Primary Care Physicians and Surgeons," *Journal of the American Medical Association* 227, no. 7 (1999): 553–59.

11. Liang, "A System of Medical Error Disclosure."

12. Web site of Lowell General Hospital: http://www.lowellgeneral.org.

13. E. G. Meinberg and P. J. Stern, "Incidence of Wrong-Site Surgery Among Hand Surgeons," *The Journal of Bone & Joint Surgery, Inc.* 85, no. 2 (2003): 193–97.

14. Author interview with Dr. Nicholas Masi, director of family-centered care at the Joe DiMaggio Children's Hospital, Fort Lauderdale, Florida, May 2, 2003.

15. T. L. Leaman and J. W. Saxton, *Preventing Malpractice: The Coactive Solution* (New York: Plenum Publishing Co., 1993).

16. T. L. Leaman and J. W. Saxton, *Managed Care Success: Reducing Risk While Increasing Patient Satisfaction* (Frederick, Md.: Aspen Publishers, Inc., 1998), 195.

17. Ibid.

18. Ibid., 201.

19. D. S. Main and others, "Patient Perspective on the Doctor of the Future," *Family Medicine* 34, no. 4 (2002): 251–57.

20. M. B. Kapp, "Medical Error versus Malpractice," *DePaul Journal of Health Care Liability* 1 (Summer 1997): 751, 752; see also L. Gostin, "A Public Health Approach to Reducing Error: Medical Malpractice as a Barrier," *Journal of the American Medical Association* 283, no. 13 (2000): 1742–43.

21. M. B. Kapp, "Legal Anxieties and Medical Mistakes," *Journal of General Internal Medicine* 12, no. 12 (1997): 787–88.

22. A. B. Witman, D. M. Park, and S. B. Hardin, "How Do Patients Want Physicians to Handle Mistakes? A Survey of Internal Medicine Patients in an Academic Setting," *Archives of Internal Medicine* 156 (1996): 2565–69.

23. A. W. Wu, "Handling Hospital Errors: Is Disclosure the Best Defense?" *Annals of Internal Medicine* 131 (1999): 970–72.

24. L. O. Prager, "New Laws Let Doctors Say 'I'm Sorry' for Medical Mistakes," *American Medical News* (2000) (http://www.ama-assn.org/sci-pubs/amnews/pick_00/prsa0821.htm).

25. Hickson and others, "Factors That Prompted Families to File Medical Malpractice Claims."

26. Prager, "New Laws Let Doctors Say 'I'm Sorry' for Medical Mistakes."

27. R. M. Lamb and others, "Hospital Disclosure Practices: Results of a National Survey," *Health Affairs* 22, no. 2 (2003): 73–83.

28. Ibid.

29. Kraman and Hamm, "Risk Management."

30. M. Crane, "What to Say If You Made a Mistake," *Medical Economics* 78, no. 16 (2001): 26–36.
31. Kraman and Hamm, "Risk Management."
32. Veterans Health Administration, *Patient Safety Improvement* (Washington, D.C.: Department of Veterans Affairs, 1988), 1051/1.
33. Crane, "What to Say If You Made a Mistake."
34. 28 U.S.C. § 2674.
35. 42 U.S.C. §§ 11101 *et seq.* (The Health Care Quality Improvement Act of 1986).
36. Kraman and Hamm, "Risk Management."
37. Wu, "Handling Hospital Errors."
38. See *State Farm Mutual Automobile Ins. Co. v. Campbell*, 538 U.S. __, 123 S. Ct. 1513; 155 L. Ed. 2d 585 (2003).
39. Lamb, "Hospital Disclosure Practices," 76.
40. Hickson and others, "Factors That Prompted Families to File Medical Malpractice Claims."
41. Liang, "Error in Medicine."
42. Kraman and Hamm, "Risk Management."
43. American Society for Healthcare Risk Management, *Perspective on Disclosure of Unanticipated Outcome Information* (Chicago: ASHRM, April 2001).
44. Ibid.
45. Leaman and Saxton, *Managed Care Success,* 133; see also Wu, "Handling Hospital Errors."
46. C. Johnson and S. Horton, "Owning Up to Errors; Put an End to the Blame Game," *Nursing* (June 2001): 54.
47. 45 C.F.R. §§ 160 & 164.
48. 45 C.F.R. § 164.510(b)(1)(i)
49. 45 C.F.R. § 164.510(b)(2)(i)–(iii).
50. 45 C.F.R. § 160.202.

6

Call to Action:
The Leader's Role in Patient Safety

Thomas C. Royer, M.D.

The goal of excellent patient care is either explicitly expressed or clearly implied in the mission, vision, and value statements of most health care institutions today. To attain this goal, leadership must "walk the talk" and create an environment and culture where strides to achieve excellence are made every day. Our leadership training teaches excellence, our practitioners strive for it, and our patients and their families deserve it. Leaders of the health delivery process have the responsibility and therefore must be accountable to ensure that the highest quality of care is being delivered to each and every person who enters our doors.

Although creating the vision for excellence may at first seem easy, bringing it to fruition requires a great deal of effort. One explanation is that neither the public nor practicing physicians have a sense of urgency about patient safety and medication errors, according to numerous studies. This is a concern of many national consumer activist organizations. In fact, according to one recent survey, neither physicians nor the public consider medical errors a significant problem in health care today.[1]

Role of Health Care Leaders

So how do health care leaders make excellence a reality? Hospital CEOs and medical directors should take an active interest in patient safety initiatives and support efforts to engage physicians, associate staff, patients, and families in the process. Focused and constant attention is the currency of leadership. Many people will follow if leaders make safety walk-arounds, endorse nonpunitive reporting, and work with the medical executive committee to address issues of poor physician performance. In addition, leadership must encourage open, candid conversations about safety, not only with staff at all levels of the organization, but with patients and their families as well. This feedback can be obtained during "real-time" rounds or, retrospectively, with randomly chosen focus groups. Possible questions to ask in these focus groups would include the following:

- Are all caregivers identifying themselves to you?
- Is each person you encounter explaining what he or she is trying to do with you?
- Do you feel a trust or confidence in your caregivers?
- Are there times when you have not felt safe? When?
- Would you recommend these services to a friend?
- What could we do to make you feel more secure?

The information received and the suggestions made should be broadly communicated and become a part of the planning process so that appropriate corrective action plans can be put into place.

Consistent Communication

Both verbal and written communications articulated often and consistently must be utilized to elevate patient safety to its appropriate level of importance. This can be accomplished through internal communications to staff members and physicians as well as to patients, using patient education materials or information placed in hospital billing statements. To promote accountability, measurable goals for each of these tactics should be developed and included in annual performance appraisal goals. These should, in part, drive any annual merit increase and also be integrated into any incentive or pay-at-risk programs available to leadership teams. In addition, these communication activities should be incorporated into the organization's annual strategic planning goals. Examples of such strategies would include the following:

- Patient safety activities are identified and implemented in all departments and facilities.
- Education materials to facilitate employee focus on improving patient safety are developed and incorporated into the orientation program for new employees.
- A patient safety suggestion box for patients and families is placed in a high-traffic area in both inpatient and outpatient facilities.

Strategic Planning

An effective strategic planning effort allows health care leadership and their staffs to design and implement a solid medication safety and patient safety plan. It is imperative that a risk assessment first be done to identify areas where process improvement is needed. Patients and families should be included in these assessments, with input obtained through follow-up phone calls or brief written surveys. Information obtained from such follow-ups in my organization has included the following:

- No one checked my armband before I was given medication.
- A puddle of water on my floor was not cleaned quickly.
- I did not have the opportunity to ask questions of the caregiver before a procedure was done.
- No one explained clearly what the medication I was given was supposed to do.

The information obtained from follow-ups is used to identify specific issues that will need to be incorporated into strategic goals and operating initiatives with clearly defined timelines and responsibilities.

Governance Oversight

Ultimately, accountability for not-for-profit health care delivery systems and public for-profits lies in the governance process. The organization's board of directors should have responsibility for quality oversight and either directly or indirectly (for example, as part of a quality committee) evaluate patient safety data on a regular basis. The board should likewise monitor patient involvement by assessing patient satisfaction scores at least quarterly.

Patient safety measurements should be included in the board's quality report. These measures should be identical to those being reviewed on a regular basis by management to determine if management is meeting its patient satisfaction goals. Clearly, the board report, at a minimum, should include the following:

- Medication errors
- Wrong-site surgeries
- Near miss incidents
- Falls
- Puncture/needle wounds
- Equipment failures

But more important than identifying the "failures" is to clearly articulate what action plans are being implemented to prevent errors from recurring in the future.

Operational Tactics

Clearly, excellence in patient safety will only be achieved if plans are implemented to achieve measurable outcomes within a set period. These operational tactics, which must be strongly supported by leadership, include a wide variety of approaches that can be customized to the individual organization. The most helpful include creating champions, sharing data, developing incentives for patient involvement, education, and supporting external evaluation.

Creating Champions

First and foremost, "champions" must be identified. These are credible, well-respected individuals who clearly understand the issues and possess sufficient energy and focus to lead the corrective action planning and implementation process. Patient safety improvement responsibilities should be incorporated into the job description of these champion staff members. Appropriate educational courses must be offered to expand the patient safety knowledge of the champions. In addition, networks in which they can share and develop best practices should be created.

A patient safety advisory council is most beneficial in helping the operational champions identify issues and find solutions. Membership on this advisory council should be multidisciplinary, consisting primarily of patients and consumers. The council's activities must be supported by an information technology infrastructure and focus on all patient safety concerns, including the common errors that occur when patients are transferred from one area of the continuum of care to another. This group should review and recommend technology that can minimize errors and near misses and also define data sets that can be audited periodically to verify that continuous improvement is occurring. The goal is to achieve consistent and predictable clinical performance for *all* patients at all times.

Sharing Data

Once the data are known, they should be shared internally and externally with appropriate staff, quality-focused organizations, and monitoring agencies. Voluntary peer reporting is important to determine best practices as well as to understand the gap between where an organization is presently and where it should be. Once this gap is understood, appropriate tactics must be put in place to achieve excellence. Networking among those with better performance is an ideal way to learn about, and then transplant, practices to make improvements in a "rapid cycle" fashion. In addition, all patients must have access and "ownership" of their own health data, which, it is hoped, will increase their participation in maintaining health.

Developing Incentives for Patient Involvement

It is also appropriate to develop incentives, both monetary and otherwise, to heighten patients' participation in medication safety and standardization of care. These might include rewards for compliance with drug regimens and disease management programs. Rewards should include products that are health related; successful examples include the following:

- Car seats for children
- Free or discounted physical exams
- Discounts on vitamins
- Free or discounted childhood immunizations
- Sessions in exercise clubs
- Free classes on nutrition
- Free classes on smoking cessation

Educating Patients, Families, and Staff

The leadership team should also be supportive of the development of educational programs that highlight ways that patients and their families can collaborate with caregivers to ensure a safe health care environment, processes, and procedures. Patients should be encouraged to ask questions, compiled beforehand, and providers should listen carefully and answer them. Patients should also be encouraged to bring all medications to the encounter as well as a copy of their advance directive. Any instructions, including information about medications, should be given in the language a patient can understand, and prescription labeling should be clear and distinct.

While in the hospital, patients should receive constant reminders to make sure all members of their caregiver team are aware of patients' important personal health information, such as allergies or chronic conditions. Also, patients should feel free to question medication and tests as they would in an outpatient setting. All of this information is extremely helpful and can be included in a patient guidebook.

The guidebook would remind patients to actively participate in ensuring their own safety. Patients should be encouraged to ask all caregivers if they are familiar with patients' allergies and the combination of medicines patients are taking. Patients should also be made aware of major safety hazards, such as not having assistance when medicated, falling over equipment cluttering the space around the bed, or being asked to take medicine left at the bedside. A whiteboard in each patient's room, where the patient, family, and caregivers can easily view it, is also an excellent method of recording data to enhance the safety environment for the patient.

The name of the major caregivers by shift, as well as the patient's allergies, should be clearly available to all caregivers coming to the bedside. The patient's chronic conditions and medications can also be included on the board; but in light of HIPAA privacy regulations, the patient's consent must first be given. The more this type of information is consistently available, the safer the environment will be.

Supporting External Evaluation

Although at times challenging, health care leaders should also support external accrediting bodies that survey any aspect of patient safety. The findings of such surveys may contain some controversial issues at times, but this feedback provides one more set of eyes to evaluate performance, identify gaps between reality and goals, and offer advice for improvement. The continuous improvement mentality that the outside review process creates in a facility is a positive halo effect in moving the organization to a higher level of patient safety and improved quality.

Making Excellence Commonplace

Health care leaders carry an awesome responsibility, because patients entering our doors are placing their life—their most precious gift—in our hands. Consequently, we must strive to care for each person in an excellent manner, ensuring that the treatment environment is as safe as possible. By collaborating with patients, families, and staff and listening to suggestions, the leadership team can make continual improvements, which is why it is imperative to tap into the insightful perspectives and creative solutions of our stakeholders. More often than not, the information gleaned proves to be a valuable resource in improving safety and reducing medication errors, thereby improving the overall quality and outcome of care. In the end, we should be so confident in our ability to provide a truly safe environment—one in which excellence is commonplace—that we could offer a service guarantee to each person who walks through our doors. Otherwise, we should "pay the penalty" and rapidly institute a corrective action plan so we will achieve success in the future.

A "service guarantee" environment demands a strong team effort from staff, as well as an intense focus on getting patients and their families involved as additional safeguards in the system. Patients must be involved in education processes focusing on patient safety issues in their encounters, readily accepted as active participants in maintaining their safety during their encounters, and questioned after their encounters to understand what made them feel safe and then listen to their suggestions as to what improvements could be made. Specific examples of how to accomplish these goals are highlighted in this chapter.

On an ongoing basis, the progress in improving the health care environment so that it is providing cost-efficient and effective care delivered with the highest degree of safety possible can be monitored by periodically receiving and reviewing the following information at both the management and governance levels:

- Patient satisfaction scores
- Associate and employee satisfaction scores
- Physician satisfaction scores
- The medication error rate
- Near miss incidents
- Measurements of agreed-on quality metrics
- Patient falls
- Complaints
- Legal/risk claims
- Puncture wounds from needles
- Equipment failures
- Nosocomial infections

Every health care organization must have clearly articulated, measurable goals for patient safety. Goal attainment should be regularly monitored so that continuous improvement can be made toward creating a safe and pleasant environment for each patient who enters our doors.

Reference

1. R. J. Blendon and others, "Views of Practicing Physicians and the Public on Medical Errors," *New England Journal of Medicine* 347, no. 24 (2002): 1965–67.

7

Royal Oak Beaumont Hospital: Putting the Patient in Patient Safety

*Kay Beauregard, R.N., M.S.A.,
and Steven Winokur, M.D.*

R oyal Oak Beaumont Hospital in Royal Oak, Michigan, is a large (997 beds) community teaching hospital and a member of the AAMC Council of Teaching Hospitals. It is also a member of Beaumont Hospitals, a two-hospital system in southeast Michigan. Recently, Beaumont ranked first in the nation for inpatient hospital admissions and second nationally for total surgeries performed. Beaumont has received recognition for its performance as one of the nation's top hospitals (*U.S. News & World Report,* July 1998, 1999, 2000, 2002). Given its high volume of patients, it is essential that Beaumont do all it can to ensure patient safety. Each patient (and family/support group) plays a vital role in safe care by taking an active and informed part.

Laying the Groundwork

The Beaumont board of directors has always made patient safety a top priority. By adopting a performance improvement plan in 2000, the board of directors identified patient safety as the guiding principle in achieving quality. The board demonstrates support for patient safety through executive appointments, sufficient personnel, requests for patient safety outcome information, and resource allocation. In January 2001, Beaumont established its Patient Safety Council. The council, composed of corporate, medical staff, and quality leaders and the Department of Legal Affairs, oversees all patient safety activities. The board of directors appointed a physician leader as chief patient safety officer in 2001.

The organization's leadership demonstrates that patient safety is a top priority by communicating with employees and medical staff at all levels, encouraging active involvement of staff and physicians on patient safety committees, and educating employees about safety-related issues. The revised employee orientation program includes patient safety, and department managers' meetings routinely include items that relate to patient safety.

The sheer size of the hospital and scope of the patient safety program created a challenge in reaching all medical staff and employees. Implementing change throughout all levels of the organization required a unique blend of committed leadership, networking, and empowerment of patient safety advocates throughout the organization. Complex organizational theory has been extremely helpful in designing the approach to changing our culture.

A Supportive Culture

Beaumont has a long-standing tradition of pursuit of clinical excellence, quality improvement, and outcomes measurement. Commitment to education includes training programs in the following areas:

- Graduate medical education
- Medical student education with formal medical school affiliations
- Nursing education
- Pharmacy education
- Radiology education

Beaumont is integrating the culture of safety through its leadership, education and training programs, allocation of resources, and personnel sufficient to ensure a state-of-the-art capability for process improvement.

Reporting is promoted by offering multiple paths by which participants can report an error or near miss, including written variance reports or an anonymous hotline. A nonpunitive environment for error reporting is demonstrated by the responses to reported errors. Process owners (recipients of variance reports) send thank-you letters to staff or physicians who have reported errors. Recognition programs, such as "WOW" cards, are given to staff members who participate in patient safety rounds. WOW cards are the size of a business card and are redeemable for hospital dining room and gift shop discounts.

The human resources department provides education and support to managers for ensuring that staff involved in errors have appropriate assistance and are not penalized. Counseling and support services are available to all employees and medical staff who might need to overcome feelings of grief, frustration, anger, embarrassment, guilt, or loss of confidence that may occur as a result of clinical error. Incorporating "patient safety story telling" has been effective in promoting candid discussion. Staff members who see genuine process change as a result of their reports will continue to report.

Process improvement teams composed of process owners develop and implement risk reduction action plans to prevent recurrences of similar events. Action plans are continually evaluated for effectiveness based on data. Patients are asked to provide feedback regarding patient safety. Specific instructions are given to patients on partnering with caregivers to provide safe care. Patients and families have a dedicated phone line on which to report safety concerns, and they learn about the phone line from printed material, such as the "Partners in Safety" brochure that is described later in this chapter. The phone line is the same one publicized in the bedside patient guide and other informational brochures for dealing with patient concerns. The phone line connects patients to the customer relations department, whose personnel handle calls promptly and involve the unit manager and other appropriate personnel. Although the phone line is available for use during the hospital stay, many patients and families prefer to call after discharge.

Policies That Form the Foundation

Various policies were developed or revised to support the patient safety infrastructure and reflect patient safety as our guiding principle in achieving quality. Policies support such concepts as recognition of human errors as inevitable, even among the most conscientious professionals practicing the highest standard of care, and recognition that learning from errors is critical if we are to design safer systems. These policies cover topics such as variance reporting, sentinel event response, and corrective actions.

The chain-of-command policy describes the expectation that staff will report real or potential patient safety issues and the infrastructure to support staff when they do. The informed consent policy describes the expectation that patients will be involved in decision making. A new policy, called "Employees Involved in Clinical Errors" was developed to encourage a patient-safe culture. The policy outlines the support process, which is intended to assist employees in resolving such issues as grief, frustration, embarrassment, and so on when they are involved in a clinical error. These policies provide a consistent framework from which all departments can function. They demonstrate a commitment to staff members that the organization will support them as individual practitioners and will focus on providing systems that promote safe care for the patient.

The Impact of Change

The culture change at Beaumont has been observable in a number of different ways, such as the following:

- An increase in error reporting has been documented, including an increase in the reporting of close-call events.
- Discussions of patient safety issues occur at staff meetings on a regular basis.
- Nurses routinely read back orders to physicians.
- Transporters "stop the line" and don't take patients off the unit without an identification band physically attached to all patients.

Processes have changed as a direct result of analysis and prioritization of variance report data by process owners. The medication process owner and his team developed a targeted intervention to improve the clarity and completeness of the approximately 3,000 written medication orders received each day by the pharmacy. Seven specific guidelines were developed for medication order writing. Medications could not be dispensed or administered until the order complied with these guidelines, at times requiring the order be rewritten by the physician.

In a two-week educational campaign, physicians, nurses, unit secretaries, respiratory therapists, and pharmacists were trained in the new medication-ordering process. The campaign involved 60 in-service training sessions, along with 700 posters, 2,000 fliers, 200 buttons, and 2,000 pocket cards. This campaign resulted in a 24 percent overall improvement in the completeness of medication orders. The impact of the resulting change demonstrated the concept of shared accountability for the medication process, and the project reinforced to the staff that leadership is committed to process improvement. Understanding that safety is about process improvement and not finding someone to blame leads to a more open culture. This open culture is necessary if physicians and staff members are to feel comfortable (and safe) inviting patients to participate in the care process.

Current Strengths in Patient Involvement

Beaumont has created a firm foundation of patient safety that has allowed the increased involvement of patients. Several initiatives, described in the following sections, are under way to strengthen and expand this involvement.

Patient Education Specialists

The hospital has an educational design department and dedicated education specialists who are accomplished in designing patient education materials that are translated into multiple languages and are adaptable to many situations. The educational design department has developed diverse patient education materials for specific disease categories, equipment use, and therapies; the pain scale, for example, is translated into 21 languages.

The department designs communication tools that can be used by family or health care workers to communicate with non-English-speaking or aphasic patients; patient tools are pictures and other methods to enhance communication. Enhanced communication with patients and families results in a greater chance of a safer outcome. During the patient identification process, for example, patients are asked to state their name; to ensure that staff can adequately communicate with all patients, this request has been translated into Arabic (figure 7-1).

Recognition of Patient Involvement

The hospital embraces and fosters cultural diversity. Interpreter services are available, as are a large number of clinical pathways, clinical practice guidelines, and patient pathways. Patient versions of pathways help to foster patient safety; these pathways describe for patients the tests, treatments, and therapies that can be expected during their course of stay. Patients are encouraged to question variations from the pathway—for example, if a therapy that is listed on the patient pathway for a specific postoperative day does not occur, the patient can bring this omission to the nurse's attention; or if a patient is asked to undergo a diagnostic test that is not listed on the pathway, the patient can question the deviation. Patients' actions may prevent a missed therapy or an inadvertent mistake in the

Figure 7-1.   Beaumont Hospitals Patient Identification Request, Translated into Arabic

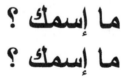

ما إسمك ؟

ما إسمك ؟

What is your name?

Source: Beaumont Hospitals, Royal Oak, Michigan, 2003. Reprinted with permission.

ordering process that could cause a patient to undergo an incorrect diagnostic test.

Inviting Patients to Participate

Efforts to include patients as partners on the health care team include development of a brochure titled "You and Your Caregivers: Partners in Safety." Educational specialists, public relations specialists, physicians, nurses, and other leaders came together to develop a brochure that communicates to patients how they can participate in their own care. It conveys that patients have a role in making health care safe and that patient safety is a top priority for us. The brochure gives the patient specific directions on how to participate in his or her care, such as through the patient identification process, medication process, surgical process, infection control, and other safety tips. Contents of the brochure are found in figure 7-2.

The brochure is included in the packet of information that patients receive on admission and are also mailed to patients prior to outpatient procedures. Physicians and staff members are encouraged to use the information in the brochure to open a discussion with patients about the value of the patients' involvement in care, and it assists the staff in articulating the concept of partnering with patients.

Through the brochure development process, it was discovered that the health care team had different opinions about how the patient could be involved in his or her care. Thus, it was important that implementation of the "You and Your Caregivers" brochure involved patients as well as physicians and staff. Everyone needed to expand his or her understanding of the patient's role in safety. The medical director sent an introductory letter to every physician with a copy of the brochure indicating that patients would be receiving the brochure, and hospital administration sent a similar letter to all department managers indicating that patients would be receiving the brochure—all of which demonstrated leadership support for involvement of the patient. It is expected that caregivers will view a patient's questioning care as providing an opportunity to prevent an error.

Figure 7-2.   Contents of the "You and Your Caregivers: Partners in Safety" Brochure at Beaumont Hospitals

---

Everyone has a role in making health care safe: physicians, nurses, pharmacists, technicians . . . **and even you!** Patient safety is a top priority for Beaumont Hospitals. As the patient, you also play a vital role in safe care by taking an active and informed part.

People come to Beaumont for the excellence of the care—and for the staff who provide that care. In health care, many complex medical procedures are performed daily. Please help your caregiver provide the kind of care you expect from Beaumont.

Please tell us if you have questions or concerns about your care.

- If possible, bring a family member or friend with you. That individual can help you feel more comfortable and help you remember questions you may have or instructions you receive.

- Feel free to ask questions to clarify what a medication is for, what test is going to be performed, or why something is being done.

- You're welcome to call our customer hotline: 248-551-2273

Pay attention to the care you are receiving.

- You'll be asked your name and will have your wristband ID checked often during your stay. This will help us identify who you are as we provide care.

- Make sure your nurse or doctor checks your wristband or asks your name before administering any medication or treatment.

- If you're having surgery, you can expect your doctor to mark the area that is to be operated on. Please feel free to ask about it.

- Expect health care workers to introduce themselves when they enter your room. Look for their name badges.

- Illness can spread when individuals do not wash their hands or wear gloves. It's OK to ask those who touch you whether they have washed their hands.

- Tell your nurse or doctor if something doesn't seem quite right.

Know what medications you are taking and why.

- Carry a list of *all* medications that you take and the amount you take. Include vitamins, herbal supplements and over-the-counter drugs. This information is important to your caregivers.

- Tell your doctors and nurses about any allergies, side effects, or problems you have had with medications in the past or are currently experiencing.

- We expect questions. Feel free to ask why a medication is being given or if it looks different or unusual to you.

Figure 7-2. (Continued)

Educate yourself about your diagnosis, the medical tests you are
having, and your treatment plan.

• Ask for information about your condition from your doctor or nurse.
  We often have written booklets, videos, educational TV programs,
  and information about Web sites and support groups.

• Make sure that information you will need is written down.

• Make sure you know how to use any equipment needed for your
  care at home after you leave the hospital.

Be a part of all decisions about your treatment.

• Share all information about your medical condition and any special
  needs with your caregivers.

• Be sure to provide details about your medical history, such as
  illnesses and operations, as well as symptoms you are having.

• Make sure you understand the information you receive. Ask
  questions as many times as you need to.

Source: Beaumont Hospitals, Royal Oak, Michigan, 2003. Reprinted with
permission.

As the process evolves, we are learning of more opportunities
for patients to participate in their care. For example, on patient
safety rounds in the patient registration area, leaders learned that
registration clerks have the patient review the wristband before it is
attached to confirm accuracy. Feedback from our volunteer staff
indicates that we need to have the brochure translated into different languages. Furthermore, patients have stated they think the
information is good and are pleased to see the hospital is being
proactive in its approach to safety.

Patient Interviews on Safety Rounds

Administrative and management rounds are conducted weekly by
administrators, patient safety officers, infection control practitioners, and environmental safety experts. All inpatient and ambulatory
settings, encompassing 61 departments, were visited in 2002. As
part of the rounds, the leaders discuss safety with at least one
patient to gain feedback from the patient's perspective. The "You
and Your Caregivers" brochure is used to guide the conversation,
such as by asking the following (or similar) questions:

- Have you noticed the staff asking you to state your name, or have they checked your identification band?
- Have you or your family had a chance to review the information in this brochure?
- If you had surgery, were you asked to mark your surgical site? If so, what do you think about that process?
- Would you feel comfortable asking a doctor if he or she had washed his or her hands before examining you?

The patient safety leaders also use the rounds to model or demonstrate methods for discussing safety issues with patients to assist managers in developing these skills.

Customized Patient Education Materials

The educational design department has developed a process to incorporate patient safety tips when developing materials. If the subject matter expert (author) for the educational materials has not included patient safety information, the patient education specialist will bring this to the author's attention. The authors are referred to the "You and Your Caregivers" brochure as a reference. Other resources, such as those developed by the National Patient Safety Foundation, are also used. Patient educational materials have an approval process that includes departmental, medical, and administrative involvement. For example, in the "Diabetes—What You Need to Know" educational booklet, the safety tips include these:

- Check the label on your insulin bottle to be sure you have the correct type.
- Make sure your insulin syringe and insulin bottle are marked with the same concentration.
- Always read your labels.

Active Patient Involvement

Although the goal is to have active patient involvement in health care processes, caregivers can't expect patients to intuitively know how they can be involved. It is also not expected that patients will know about health care processes or when to question the process.

Thus, caregivers are evaluating specific processes to determine how and when to invite the patient to be involved. Physicians and staff members need to prompt and direct patients on how they can be involved.

The point of involvement should be at a critical quality step—the point at which patient involvement in error prevention would be a valued addition. Patient (or family) involvement at a critical quality step adds another layer of safety. The following examples demonstrate practices where active involvement of patients in a specific process is encouraged:

- Patients are involved in the site-marking process for surgery.
- Patients are involved in the patient identification process. A patient actively states his or her first and last name instead of responding to a health care worker who calls out the name. In some instances, patients have been known to respond to an incorrect name. Recently, a patient was asked why he answered to the wrong name and the patient's comment was: "It was the right time for my test, so I thought it was me."
- Patients participate in the process of protecting children from abductions. Patients are told: "We want to prevent an abduction, and this is how you can help." This statement makes it more real to parents and has been incorporated into our written patient/family educational materials.
- Patients in the dialysis unit are asked to validate that we are using the correct (matched) dialyzer prior to a treatment.
- Patients are asked to read and verbally confirm their name and, when available, birth date on materials that are given to them. For example, they may be asked to verify their name on medical records, prescription medications, and radiology studies (X-rays).

Promoting Safety through Community Education

Beaumont has an outreach program called the School of Community Education, in which 81 courses are offered multiple times throughout each year. The number of community members participating in the courses ranges from 15,000 to 25,000 annually.

Course instructors are hospital employees, and they discuss patient safety issues with the participants. A script is provided for the instructors so that a consistent message of the hospital's patient safety philosophy is imparted to participants. The childbirth educator coordinator has given the following feedback:

> The brochure has been in our childbirth education folders since March 2003. These folders contain all class handouts for the series and are given to participants the first night of class. The instructors are reviewing the brochure during the course. I met with the instructors last week and their feedback was that the information is very pertinent to our curriculum and well received by expectant parents. We emphasize partnering with health care providers, informed decision making, and communication as very important in learning about and planning for birth and early parenting. This brochure assists in emphasizing these points.

The School of Community Education is a major effort to reach out to the community and educate people about their key role in safety.

Gaining Employee Input

To gain further insight into opportunities for involving patients in their care, employees are being asked to help. A patient safety leader assembled a cross-departmental group and facilitated a roundtable discussion. Recognizing that our employees have also been consumers of health care, we asked them: "How do you check that things are going right when you or a loved one is seeking medical care?" The answers vary.

- A phlebotomist stated, "I ask to see the blood label to verify my name when blood is being drawn, or I may ask to observe that the correct label is being put on the correct tube."
- A pharmacist responded, "I assess the medications my loved one is receiving."
- Another responded, "I read the chart, ask questions, mark procedure sites, and educate myself about my condition."

These perspectives are valuable as the organization seeks new opportunities to involve patients in their care. Although this was a one-time exercise, it can be repeated in any patient safety meeting. The exercise demonstrates to staff members that they should personally practice techniques to safeguard against errors and that there is value in teaching patients to do the same.

Gaining Patient Input

Members of the patient safety committees are encouraged to identify patients who could be invited to attend a patient safety meeting. Another source of valuable input is the hospital's volunteer staff, because volunteers visit a large percentage of patients each day. The patient safety leaders met with a large group of volunteers, educated them about the principles of patient safety, and asked for their assistance. During their rounds, volunteers are encouraged to reinforce the "You and Your Caregivers: Partners in Safety" brochure and emphasize the patient's role in patient safety, and volunteers are also invited to be advocates for patient safety.

Additional Partnership Opportunities

There are several opportunities that the hospital is currently investigating to improve patient participation in the safety movement. These include the following:

- Development of an orientation video for patients. The orientation video would show vignettes of patient involvement in safety and would also show willingness of staff to assist patients who have questions. The video would be part of the hospital's patient television system. One option under consideration is to have the program air the first time the patient watches television.

- Thirty-one different support groups currently meet at the hospital. Some support groups are for patients with chronic conditions such as diabetes, heart disease, and cancer. The hospital is exploring ways in which patient safety education can be incorporated into these support activities.

- Provide patients with Web site links to help them learn more about health care processes and their role in safety (for example, Web sites on medication use, what you need to know about anesthesia). These online learning suggestions would be provided through the hospital's consumer Web site (www.beaumonthospitals.com). The information on these Web links would help patients learn about relevant care issues before they come to the hospital.

Continuing Involvement After an Adverse Event

Because trust is paramount and a foundation of patient safety, Beaumont has an active process of disclosure of any event that results in an unanticipated outcome. Beaumont recognizes that after the disclosure the patient and/or family continue to need assistance. Support may be needed to work through an anger or grief process or to understand what the hospital has done to prevent future occurrences; pastoral care and social work departments may become actively involved in these situations.

Measuring Success

Evaluating the achievement of patient safety goals is accomplished through direct feedback from frontline care providers, support staff, and patients. Patient safety leaders use patient safety rounds to gather feedback from staff about the effectiveness of the program. Departmental patient safety assessment tools are provided for managers to use in assessing implementation of patient safety interventions.

Beaumont also conducts organizationwide employee and physician surveys to assess patient safety culture, teamwork, error reporting (nonpunitive environment), education, and leadership responsiveness to patient safety issues. The types of information that are gleaned from these surveys are illustrated in figure 7-3. Areas for improvement are identified and assigned to key leaders in the organization. Progress toward resolution is tracked through the hospital's performance improvement structure. Patient safety measures are reported monthly to the board.

Figure 7-3.   Results of Employee Patient Safety Surveys at Beaumont Hospitals

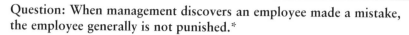

Question: When management discovers an employee made a mistake, the employee generally is not punished.*

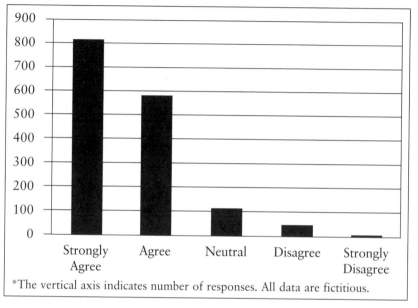

*The vertical axis indicates number of responses. All data are fictitious.

Question: When I or someone in my work area makes a mistake, we should all know about it so others don't make the same mistake.*

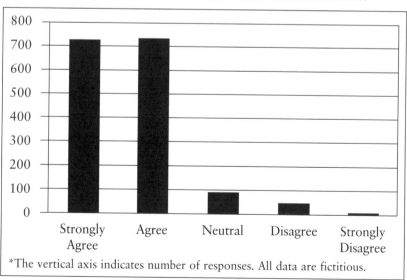

*The vertical axis indicates number of responses. All data are fictitious.

Source: Beaumont Hospitals, Royal Oak, Michigan, 2003. Reprinted with permission.

Patient Satisfaction Survey

The hospital utilizes a standard patient satisfaction survey process. A vendor is used to mail out approximately 100 surveys per day to previously discharged patients. The return rate is about 40 percent. Specific questions relating to patient safety included the following:

- Did the health care worker spend sufficient time reviewing your admission packet?
- Did you feel appropriately involved in your care?
- If there were any unplanned or unanticipated events in your care, were you kept informed in a timely and satisfactory manner?

These questions are part of the overall survey process, the results of which are analyzed by the patient satisfaction council.

Department Data on Patient Safety

A patient safety department assessment tool is used during patient safety rounds (figure 7-4). Managers complete this self-assessment of patient safety efforts within their department. Data are aggregated on each question. Questions specific to patient/family communication include the following:

- Patients are included in safety planning by encouraging them to participate in their care.
- Written materials are provided to patients and families that describe their role as partners in patient safety.
- The department embraces its responsibility and acknowledges its ethical obligation to communicate with patients when unanticipated outcomes have occurred. This includes an explanation of the outcome and its effects, provided in a timely, truthful, and compassionate manner.

Other questions focus on department leadership, creating a learning environment, teamwork and collaboration, and performance measurement.

Figure 7-4.   Royal Oak Beaumont Hospital Patient Safety Department Assessment

Place an "X" in the box that most closely represents implementation status.

A = fully implemented throughout the department
B = partially implemented in the department
C = discussed but not implemented
D = no activity

Key Aspect of Safety: Leadership	A	B	C	D
Patient safety goals and objectives are communicated across the department.				
Department leadership regularly monitors and communicates progress in implementing the patient safety initiatives/programs.				
Safety principles are considered when designing and maintaining products/programs/processes.				
Department leaders establish visible commitment to patient safety by participating/performing one or more of the following activities: • Periodic observation of routine operations				
• Periodic "walkarounds" to discuss patient safety and patient safety issues with direct care providers				
Patient safety orientation is provided to all new employees/physicians.				
Employee and medical staff roles and responsibilities in advancing patient safety are appropriately included in job descriptions, orientation, and continuing education.				
Key Aspect of Safety: Creating a Learning Environment	A	B	C	D
The department complies with a nonpunitive policy to address patient adverse events involving medical staff and employees.				
Lessons learned, safe practices, insights, and alerts received from internal and external sources are evaluated and appropriately acted on.				
Recognition and reporting of errors and hazardous conditions are encouraged and rewarded by the department.				
There is a department system of feedback of information about errors and close calls that results in changes and improvements to procedures and/or systems.				
Following a patient safety adverse event, support is provided to involved staff.				

(Continued on next page)

Figure 7-4. (Continued)

Place an "X" in the box that most closely represents implementation status.

A = fully implemented throughout the department
B = partially implemented in the department
C = discussed but not implemented
D = no activity

Key Aspect of Safety: Teamwork and Collaboration	A	B	C	D
The department uses checklists, protocols, reminders, and decision support and standardizes equipment, forms, times, and locations to avoid reliance on memory.				
Patient care processes use a minimum number of steps and handoffs.				
Accurate and timely information including clinical results and reference material is available to each clinical decision maker at the point of care.				
Process redesigns and system changes are monitored for effectiveness.				
The department seeks active input from end users of technologies, supplies, and products prior to purchase.				
Interdisciplinary team training, including physicians, is routinely conducted for caregivers.				
Key Aspect of Safety: Patient/Family Communication	A	B	C	D
Patients are included in safety planning by encouraging them to participate in their care.				
Written materials are provided to patients/families that describe their role as partners in patient safety.				
The department embraces its responsibility and acknowledges its ethical obligation to communicate with patients when unanticipated outcomes have occurred. This includes an explanation of the outcome and its effects, provided in a timely, truthful, and compassionate manner.				
Key Aspect of Safety: Measurement	A	B	C	D
Performance outcomes and indicators are established to support and monitor implementation of patient safety plans and measure safety performance.				

Source: Beaumont Hospitals, Royal Oak, Michigan, 2003. Reprinted with permission.

Hospital Data on Patient Safety

The hospital has a robust system for collecting data about, and analyzing key processes through, our variance reporting structure (known as incident reports in other organizations). Specific problematic processes were initially selected by analyzing historical data about variances. Once the key processes of interest were determined (patient falls, medication events, equipment events, and so on), process owners were recruited. A management engineer, an administrator, and a physician provide support for each process owner.

A standardized system was developed for all process owners to use in assessing, tracking, and analyzing variance data. All process owners evaluate events using a predefined set of potential root-cause process breakdowns. Root-cause process breakdowns include security systems and processes, the physical environment, equipment, patient identification process, and so on. Data from all process owner reports are aggregated, so the organization can see improvement opportunities in individual processes as well as opportunities that cross process lines. The information is used to establish safety improvement priorities for the organization. A sample aggregate report of process breakdowns is shown in figure 7-5.

As with any continuous process improvement effort, Beaumont focuses actions on the opportunities identified. The overall results of the patient safety survey show that through employee education programs we are attaining our goal of reinforcing systems to minimize errors, learning from our mistakes, and sharing what we have learned with others while keeping the patient at the center of all we do.

Specific measurement of the impact of patient involvement on error reduction will be difficult to extrapolate from existing data. Patient involvement adds one more safety layer to reduce the risk of errors; thus, the actual events should decrease. The process of patient involvement can be measured through direct observations (for example, did the staff member ask the patient to state his or her name?). To evaluate the impact of the actual involvement, staff members may be encouraged to report (through existing variance report systems) instances where the patient's involvement prevented an error.

Figure 7-5. Report of Process Breakdowns Contributing to Variances at Beaumont Hospitals*

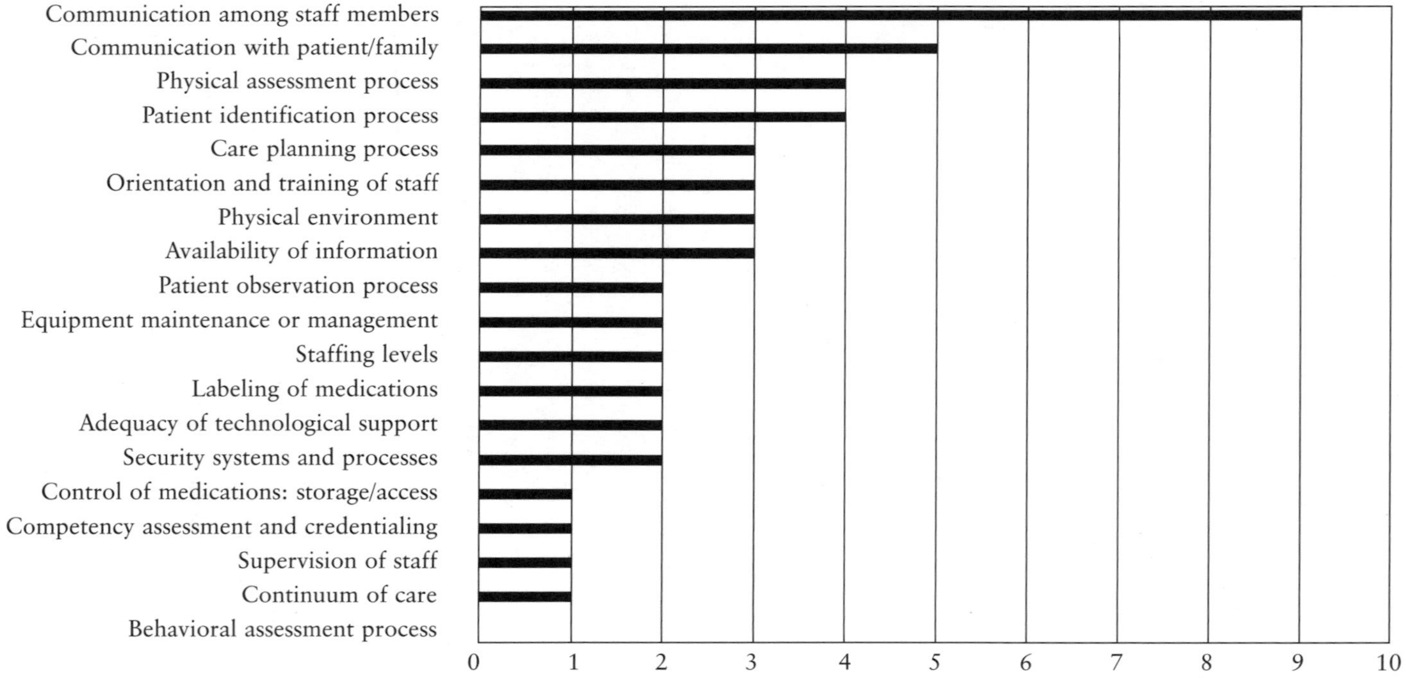

*The horizontal axis indicates the number of reported breakdowns. All data are fictitious.

Source: Beaumont Hospitals, Royal Oak, Michigan, 2003. Reprinted with permission.

The Patient as Partner in Safe Care

It is essential for health care organizations to create a culture of patient safety before jumping in with the expectation that staff will embrace patients as partners in care. The fundamentals of building safe systems, process improvement, learning from errors and close calls, and reducing the fear of inappropriate punitive reactions will build a culture of trust. Staff members who are equipped with the appropriate skills and practice in a supportive culture will more readily embrace the value of having the patient as a partner in care. Organizations that are proactive and teach patients how to be partners in the patient safety movement will have a win-win situation.

Resource List

Numerous resources are available to help patients and their families participate more fully in the health care experience. Below are resources specifically focused on engaging consumers in patient safety. Some of the materials are intended to educate consumers on their role in reducing medical errors, and other resources are for health care professionals seeking ways to improve consumer involvement in safety initiatives. Many of the organizations and companies listed have additional health care quality and safety improvement resources. The number of resources that can be used to engage consumers in patient safety continues to grow every day. A current list of resources is maintained on the Internet at: http://www.brownspath.com/safecare.htm.

Health Care Safety Fact Sheets and Other Resources for Consumers

Agency for Healthcare Research and Quality
http://www.ahrq.gov

Consumer fact sheets and brochures (some Spanish versions):

- 20 Tips to Help Prevent Medical Errors
- 5 Steps to Safer Health Care
- Your Guide to Choosing Quality Health Care
- Questions to Ask Your Doctor Before You Have Surgery
- Improving Health Care Quality: A Guide for Patients and Families
- Ways You Can Help Your Family Prevent Medical Errors
- 20 Tips to Help Prevent Medical Errors in Children

American Academy of Osteopaedic Surgeons
http://orthoinfo.aaos.org

Consumer fact sheets and other resources:

- Avoiding an Epidemic of Errors
- Getting the Most Out of a Visit with Your Doctor
- Partner with Physician for Best Surgical Outcome
- Patients Have Important Role in Safer Health Care
- Twelve Steps to a Safer Hospital Stay
- Patient Safety Is No Accident (bookmark)
- Essential Advice: Helping Your Doctors Do Their Best for You (audio)

Association of periOperative Nurses
http://patientsafetyfirst.org

Consumer fact sheets:

- Who's Who in the Hospital
- Finding Surgical Information You Can Trust
- Choosing a Doctor to Do Your Surgery
- What You Need to Know about Your Surgery
- What You Need to Know about Anesthesia
- Advice for Patients Concerned about Correct Site Surgery

Australian Council for Safety and Quality in Health Care
http://www.safetyandquality.org

Consumer brochure:

- 10 Tips For Safer Health Care: What Everyone Needs to Know

Council on Family Health
http://www.cfhinfo.org

Consumer fact sheets and brochures (Spanish versions available):

- Interactive Drug Facts: Medicine Label
- Ten Guides to Proper Medicine Use
- Drug Interactions: What You Should Know
- Tips for Seniors on Safe Medication Use
- Did You Know . . . ? Focus: Preventing Drug Interactions

Food and Drug Administration
http://www.fda.gov

Consumer fact sheets: (Spanish versions available)

- Drug Interactions: What You Should Know
- We Want You to Know about X-Rays: Get the Picture on Protection
- How to Give Medicine to Children
- Medicines and Older Adults
- Use Medicine Safely
- Buying Medicines and Medical Products Online

Health Consumers' Council of Western Australia
http://www.hcc-wa.asn.au

Consumer fact sheets:

- Consumer Questions to Ask about Your Discharge Planning
- Questions to Ask Your Doctor

Hospital & Healthsystem Association of Pennsylvania
http://www.haponline.org

Consumer brochures:

- Partners in Quality: Taking an Active Role in Your Health Care
- What We Do to Assure Quality Care

Institute for Safe Medication Practices
http://www.ismp.org

Consumer fact sheets:

- Be an Informed Consumer
- How You Can Help Ensure Your Safety When Receiving Cancer Treatments
- Treat Medication Samples with Respect
- Doctors Office (medication safety)
- Medication Errors That Have Occurred and How You Can Avoid Them (updated regularly)

Johns Hopkins Hospital Patient Safety Brochure
http://www.hopkinsmedicine.org/patient_safety.cfm

Joint Commission on Accreditation of Healthcare Organizations
http://www.jcaho.org

Consumer fact sheets and brochures:

- Preventing Wrong-Site Surgery
- Speak Up: Help Prevent Errors in Your Care

Madison (Wis.) Patient Safety Collaborative
http://www.madisonpatientsafety.org

Consumer fact sheets and brochures:

- Using Your Medications Safely: A Guide to Prescription Health
- Pocket Card to Record Medications
- What You Can Do to Make Healthcare Safer: A Consumer Tip Sheet
- Pharmacy Safety & Service—What You Should Expect
- How You Can Help Prevent Infections
- The Role of the Patient Advocate
- Safety as You Go from Hospital to Home

Massachusetts Coalition for the Prevention of Medical Errors
http://www.macoalition.org

Consumer brochure:

- Your Role in Safe Medication Use

Minnesota Alliance for Patient Safety
http://www.mhhp.com

Consumer brochure:

- Patient Safety: Your Role

National Center for Injury Prevention and Control
http://www.cdc.gov/ncipc

Consumer fact sheets:

- Falls and Hip Fractures among Older Adults
- Check for Safety: A Home Fall Prevention Checklist
  for Older Adults

National Council on Patient Information and Education
http://www.talkaboutrx.org

Consumer fact sheets and other education resources (some
Spanish versions):

- Your Medicine: Play It Safe
- Get the Most from Your Medicine: Managing Side Effects
- Get the Answers (wallet card)
- Prescription for Safety (mirror sticker)
- Medicine: Before You Take It, Talk about It
- Alcohol and Medicine: Ask Before You Mix
- Buying Prescription Medicines Online
- Taking the Mystery Out of Managing Your Medicines
  (video)

National Patient Safety Foundation
http://www.npsf.org

Consumer fact sheets and other education resources:

- You Can Help Improve Patient Safety
- Preventing Infections in the Hospital—What You as a Patient Can Do
- Patient Safety: Your Role in Making Healthcare Safer (video)
- What You Can Do to Make Health Care Safer
- Safety as You Go from Hospital to Home
- Pharmacy Safety and Service—What You Should Expect
- Role of the Patient Advocate
- Think It Through: A Guide to Managing the Benefits and Risks of Medicine

Society for Healthcare Consumer Advocacy
of the American Hospital Association
http://www.shca-aha.org/

Consumer brochure:

- Taking Charge of Your Healthcare

Virginians Improving Patient Care and Safety
http://www.vipcs.org/index.htm

Consumer fact sheets and brochures:

- Be Involved in Your Health Care: Tips to Help Prevent Medical Errors (Spanish version available)
- Tips on preventing medical errors related to medicines, hospital stays, surgery, home health, and other health services

Government and Not-for-Profit Groups

American Society for Healthcare Risk Management
of the American Hospital Association
http://www.ashrm.org

A professional society for health care risk management professionals and those responsible for the process of making and
carrying out decisions that will promote high-quality care,
maintain a safe environment, and preserve human and financial resources in health care organizations. This organization
published the white paper *Perspective on Disclosure of
Unanticipated Outcome Information* (April 2001).

Developing Patient Partnerships
http://www.concordance.org

A United Kingdom health education charity working with
primary care organizations and the public to make the most
of health services and help people manage their health by
improving health knowledge and communication.

Foundation for Accountability (FACCT)
http://www.facct.org

FACCT's mission is to improve health care for Americans by
advocating an accountable and accessible system in which
consumers are partners in their care and help shape the
delivery of care.

Institute for Healthcare Improvement
http://www.ihi.org

A not-for-profit organization created to help lead the
improvement of health care systems to increase continuously
their quality and value. Sponsors initiatives intended to
increase the role of patients and their families in health
services.

Medicines Partnership
http://www.medicines-partnership.org

A United Kingdom organization that is working with health care organizations and practitioners to help patients achieve maximum benefit from their medicines. Sponsored the "Ask about Medicines Week" in 2003 (www.askaboutmedicines.org) and is actively involved in putting principles of concordance into practice.

National Patient Safety Agency
http://www.npsa.nhs.uk

This independent body coordinates the safety improvement efforts of all those involved in health care in the United Kingdom. Public involvement in safety improvement is a major initiative for the organization.

National Patient Safety Foundation
http://www.npsf.org

The National Patient Safety Foundation serves as a resource for individuals and organizations committed to improving the safety of patients. One of the goals of the organization is to raise public awareness about health care safety. Its *Nothing About Me, Without Me* National Agenda for Action is intended to foster patient and family participation in patient safety.

National Resource Centre for Consumer Participation in Health
http://www.participateinhealth.org.au

Australian organization that provides information on consumer feedback and participation methodologies and assists health care organizations in developing, implementing, and evaluating consumer participation methods and models.

Partnership for Patient Safety
http://www.p4ps.org

A patient-centered initiative focused on improving the safety of health care through consumer involvement and a systems approach.

Society for Healthcare Consumer Advocacy
of the American Hospital Association
http://www.shca-aha.org

The Society for Healthcare Consumer Advocacy seeks to advance health care consumer advocacy by supporting the role of professionals who represent and advocate for consumers across the health care continuum.

Patient- and Family-Centered Care Organizations

Institute for Family-Centered Care
http://www.familycenteredcare.org

The mission of the Institute for Family-Centered Care is to advance the understanding and practice of family-centered care. The institute has developed several resources for health care professionals, including an assessment tool that can be used to evaluate the degree to which the curriculum, culture, and educational approach of a medical education program is likely to foster the competencies and attitudes necessary to practice family-centered care.

Planetree
http://www.planetree.org

The Planetree Model of health care is patient centered rather than provider focused and is committed to improving medical care from the patient's perspective. It empowers patients and families through information and education and encourages "healing partnerships" with caregivers.

Consumer Groups

Parents of Infants and Children with Kernicterus
   http://www.PICKonline.org

   This organization was developed in late 2000 by a group of
   mothers of children with severe cerebral palsy resulting from
   kernicterus, a condition caused by excessive bilirubin levels
   in newborns. PICK has helped to create awareness about
   kernicterus and strategies for preventing this avoidable
   patient injury.

Patients Association
   http://www.patients-association.com

   A United Kingdom consumer group that publishes *Patient
   Voice* magazine (back issues available online) and offers advice
   to consumers on how to create better patient-practitioner
   partnerships.

P.U.L.S.E. (Persons United Limiting Substandards and Errors
in Health Care)
   http://www.pulseamerica.org

   National consumer group geared toward education and
   support. The Web sites of state groups include some
   consumer-directed medical error prevention resources.

Voice4Patients.Com
   http://www.voice4patients.com

   Intended primarily as a resource for victims of medical error,
   this organization also offers resources to consumers for learning how to become more active partners in the health care
   experience and how to prevent mistakes.

Products/Books

American Hospital Association
http://www.aha.org

- *Disclosure of Medical Errors: Demonstrated Strategy to Enhance Communication* (video) (2001), produced by the American Society for Healthcare Risk Management
- *In the Name of the Patient* (2002), produced by the Society for Healthcare Consumer Advocacy
- *The Written Word: Guidelines for Responding in Writing to Patient Concerns* (2002), by Janet Gilbert and Heidi Harrison

B & R Publishing
http://www.patientjournal.com

Publisher of a patient journal designed for hospitalized patients and their families to record important medical information, physician names, medications, tests and procedures, and so on. The journal is intended to guide the patient through a hospital stay, beginning with admittance through the diagnostic and treatment regimen and finally discharge.

Brown-Spath & Associates
http://www.brownspath.com

Video resources designed for educating patients and their families and other health care consumers about their role in health care safety.

- Staying Safe: Your Role in the Healthcare Environment
- Staying Safe: How to Talk with Your Healthcare Team

Jossey-Bass/John Wiley & Sons
http://www.josseybass.com

Books for health care professionals:

- *Communicating with Today's Patient: Essentials to Save Time, Decrease Risk, and Increase Patient Compliance* (2000), by Joanne Desmond and Lanny R. Copeland
- *Honoring Patient Preferences: A Guide to Complying with Multicultural Patient Requirements* (1999), by Anne Knights Rundle, Maria Carvalho, and Mary Robinson
- *Managing Diversity in Health Care: Proven Tools and Activities for Leaders and Trainers* (1998), by Lee Gardenswartz and Anita Rowe
- *Through the Patient's Eyes: Understanding and Promoting Patient-Centered Care* (paperback, 2002), edited by Margaret Gerteis, Susan Edgman-Levitan, Jennifer Daley, and Thomas L. Delbanco
- *Patient as Partner: The Cornerstone of Community Health Improvement* (1997), by American Organization of Nurse Executives
- *Putting Patients First: Designing and Practicing Patient-Centered Care* (2003), edited by Susan Frampton, Laura Gilpin, and Patrick Charmel
- *What Do I Say?: Communicating Intended or Unanticipated Outcomes in Obstetrics* (2003), by James R. Woods and Fay A. Rozovsky

Savard Systems
http://www.drsavard.com

The Savard System empowers patients to be their own best health advocates and provides tools for patients to become informed and involved. The system grew out of Dr. Marie Savard's three decades of experience as a medical practitioner, first as a nurse and then a general internist and primary care physician.

- *How to Save Your Own Life* (Warner Books, 2000), by Marie Savard
- *The Savard Health Record: A Six-Step System for Managing Your Healthcare* (Time-Life Books, 2000), by Marie Savard

Miscellaneous books for health care consumers available from various book retailers, including Amazon.com:

- *American Medical Association Guide to Talking to Your Doctor* (John Wiley & Sons, 2001), by the American Medical Association
- *Confessions of a Professional Hospital Patient: A Humorous First-Person Account of How to Survive a Hospital Stay and Escape with Your Life, Dignity and a Sense of Humor* (1st Books Library, 2001), by Michael A. Weiss
- *How to Get Out of the Hospital Alive: A Guide to Patient Power* (John Wiley & Sons, 1998), by Sheldon P. Blau and Elaine Fantle Shimberg
- *How to Survive Your Hospital Stay* (Center Press, 1998), by Judy Burger Crane
- *Making Informed Medical Decisions: Where to Look and How to Use What You Find* (O'Reilly & Associates, 2000), by Lucy Thomas, Nancy Oster, and Darol Joseff
- *So You're Having a Heart Cath and Angioplasty* (John Wiley & Sons, 2003), by Magnus Ohman, Gail Cox, Stephen Fort, and Victoria K. Folger
- *The Intelligent Patient's Guide to the Doctor-Patient Relationship: Learning How to Talk So Your Doctor Will Listen* (Oxford University Press, 1998), by Barbara Korsch and Caroline Harding
- *Working with Your Doctor: Getting the Healthcare You Deserve* (O'Reilly & Associates, 1998), by Nancy Keene

Index